SEX AND YOUNG PEOPLE

Sex
and
Young People

LANCE PIERSON

KINGSWAY PUBLICATIONS
EASTBOURNE

Cover design by Drummond Chapman

Printed in Great Britain for
KINGSWAY PUBLICATIONS LTD
Lottbridge Drove, Eastbourne, E. Sussex BN23 6NT by
Cox & Wyman Ltd, Reading.
Typeset by CST, Eastbourne, E. Sussex.

I dedicate this book to all who helped put together the 'Earth Invaders' programme in spring 1982, when this book was born. Especially to the dozens of teenagers who talked to me about their sexual questions and difficulties. And to Joy and Robin, the two special 'Earth Invaders' God has given me to care for.

Contents

I

Emmanuel or Emmanuelle?

Tonight We Will Fake Love

Tonight, we will
fake love together.
You my love, possess
all the essential qualities
as listed by Playboy.
You will last me for
as long as two weeks
or until such a time
as your face & figure
go out of fashion.
I will hold you close
to my Hollywood standard body,
the smell of which
has been approved
by my ten best friends
and a representative
of Lifebuoy.
I will prop my paperback
Kama Sutra
on the dressing table
& like programmed souls

we will perform
& like human beings
we will grow tired
of our artificially sweetened
diluted & ready to drink
love affairs.
Tonight, we will fake love.
Tonight we will be both
quick & silent,
our time limited,
measured out in distances
between fingers
      & pushbuttons.[1]

There are two love-gods in the world today: Emmanuel and Emmanuelle.[2] 'Emmanuel' is one of the names of Jesus; it means 'God with us'. The whole idea of this book is that God made us and understands us. If we're Christians, he shares life with us and can show us how to enjoy it. Just as the designer of a video recorder or home computer knows how to make his product work properly, so God knows what makes human nature tick, and what's best for us. And that includes sex.

You can't shock or surprise God over anything to do with sex. He invented it! And he can teach us how to understand it and handle it, so as to make life happier and richer. In short, Emmanuel-sex—sex as Jesus teaches it—is best.

Emmanuelle-sex is the exact opposite. Nowhere in life is the way the world thinks in more complete contrast with Jesus' way than in attitudes to sex. Christians and non-Christians by and large agree that murder is wrong and kindness is right.

But when it comes to sex. . . .

Emmanuel is the God-man who *died for* every-one. Emmanuelle is the goddess-woman who *lives with* anyone. They offer the choice of sexual life-style open to people today. In this book I'm trying to show you what the choice really is, to help you make up your own mind with facts and reason-able arguments in front of you. Because one thing is for sure. Emmanuelle won't present you with an open, reasonable case. She will assault your senses with a constant stream of one-sided propaganda till your judgement is impaired and you can no longer make up your own mind. She will per-suade you to do what she wants through her channels of 'sex-ploitation'.

One of these channels is films. As I expect you've already guessed, I take the name 'Emmanuelle' from the series of sex-films made in the 1970s, which reckoned to push back the boun-daries of explicitness and experimentation till they could go no further. The market was flooded with sequels: *Emmanuelle II, Black Emmanuelle, Emmanuelle goes to Hong Kong,* etc. As one critic wittily commented, each new film was not so much 'Emmanuelle *rides* again,' but 'Emmanuelle *is ridden* again—and again—and again—and again —and again—all in the same film, by men or women, singly or in combinations!'

Another channel is commercials. At one level, there is the standard gimmick of using a picture of a pretty girl to sell any product remotely con-nected with sex-appeal: perfume, stockings, drink, cars, cigars. . . . But there is a deeper level, where an advert tries to be as suggestive as it dares, deliberately titillating our sexual excitement. Displayed not so long ago in the London underground were posters advertising an overseas holiday firm. There were three photos of people frolicking in the sea, and another three blank spaces marked *'censored!'* The caption underneath read:

> What a shame some of you are under 18 or over 30. We sympathize with those either too young or too old to experience a Club 18–30 holiday. But such are the injustices of life.
>
> Besides, the kind of living we had in mind is definitely for fun-loving pleasure-seekers who want every day to be an adventure and every night one to remember.
>
> Perhaps a peek under the 'censored' stamps would give a clearer picture. That is, if the uninvited don't mind pondering over glorious, sunfilled days brimming with exciting trips, outrageous parties and discos, romantic moonlit beaches and kindred spirits to share it all with.
>
> Just choose the right background for your fantasies. . . . And take no notice of the sidelong green looks you're getting.
>
> Just remember: *No other holiday would dare.*

And there are other channels, too, including songs, books and magazines. But through them all Emmanuelle's message is pretty clear, isn't it? This is how it goes: 'The vital thing in life is to be sexy and attractive. So off with the pimples and the B.O., and on with the shampoo and conditioning cream and hair lacquer; the eye-shadow and ear-rings and after-shave lotion; the lipstick and toothpaste and underarm deodorant; and, of course, the right curve-hugging underwear. And *then* . . . you are irresistible!'

And Emmanuelle goes on: 'If two of you are attracted to each other, there is no reason in the world why you shouldn't glide into each other's arms in the course of a single evening, ending up in, well, bed preferably; or on a hearthrug, if you're in a hurry; or in a broom-cupboard, if there's nowhere else! And then you drift romantically along on cloud nine until . . . well, until you meet a yet more stupendous body; someone even more sensational and ravishing and knock-out!'

And you know what my reaction to all that is? I like the sound of it very much indeed. I wouldn't be normal if I didn't. As a twentieth-century male, I am 'extremely interested' in sex, to put it mildly, and I don't mind admitting it. Books or magazines about sex hold a strong fascination for me and lure me irresistibly to pore over them. This is simply human nature.

The real world we live in is sex-centred; some would say sex-crazed or sex-obsessed. In teenage years, when sexual feelings first explode into life and are at their peak, the subject is almost all-absorbing. To some extent this must always have been true: the young adult in any generation or society is naturally curious about how his body works, and eager to experiment with it. But thanks to Emmanuelle's propaganda campaign, sex is up on the surface, open to be talked about, read about, watched and spied upon, as never before.

13

Much of this is healthy, of course. It is thoroughly good that sex is not a forbidden subject surrounded with all sorts of black suspicions and old wives' tales any more.

Emmanuelle's lies

But there is just one snag. A lot of the buzz that Emmanuelle spreads around is just as phoney as the old Victorian myths. The Emmanuelle message is a con; it's a put-up job, a fantasy. It's full of lies, designed to deceive. Such as? Well, take a look at these, for starters.

Lie no. 1: sex is instant kicks

The Emmanuelle films give the impression that you can achieve an earth-shattering sexual climax with a complete stranger as soon as you meet them. But this is utter rubbish. The whole set-up is absurdly oversimplified. In the make-believe, 'wouldn't-it-be-nice-if' world of sex films, women are never having a period or a 'headache' or feeling too tired. Their clothes seem to slip off almost automatically, without getting caught or twisted or in the way. Men are never unsure or nervous or clumsy. Nobody experiences any discomfort. Contraceptives appear to be unnecessary (at any rate, they're never mentioned). And sexually transmitted diseases are unheard of! It's all too convenient to be true!

Alas, real life is not like that. One-third of all babies are conceived by unmarried parents, and venereal disease continues to increase, especially among teenagers, despite more widely available information and treatment.

But more fundamentally, when people ask me, as they often do, 'Why shouldn't I sleep with my boyfriend/girlfriend if I love him/her?' the answer I usually give is, 'The chances are ten-to-one that you wouldn't enjoy it.' Research among sexually experienced teenagers shows that less than half the boys and under a third of the girls even claim to have liked their first time. Common reactions were disappointment, shame or fear. 'What's all the fuss about?' asked one disillusioned eighteen-year-old girl.

The reason for this is that sexual intercourse is the expression of a relationship between two people. When they are unsure of each other, any attempt at sexual union will be uncertain, unco-ordinated and unharmonious. He will probably reach a climax (of sorts) long before he wants to and almost certainly she won't reach one at all. If you don't believe me, listen to any 'topless radio' show, when people phone in to talk to a coun-sellor about their sexual problems.

But for a couple happily married along Emmanuel lines, who are getting to know and understand each other better and better, sexual harmony and happiness will steadily grow. This is because you need time to adjust to each other, to learn each other's ways and to discover how to give each other pleasure. And that in turn takes patience, commitment and oodles of a relaxed sense of humour. The human body, with its tendency to let you down at awkward or embarrassing moments, is a bit of a clown. To Emmanuel's followers this is all part of the fun; but to Emmanuelle's devotees it's a disaster, because they are 'on display' to the current partner and have to be grimly serious as they take their 'pleasure'. One of Emmanuelle's many fallacies is to take the genuine giggle and laughter out of sex.

And she takes away the tender relaxation as well. How can you possibly be open and relaxed with your partner if he or she is not completely committed to you? The whole time you are 'on approval', wondering whether you are giving them the blinding sensation they expect of you, or whether you will be ditched in the morning because you didn't perform well enough.

This is where the hideous 'one standard for men and another for women' comes from. Emmanuelle gives men the 'easy lay' they want, and so betrays her own sex. They tell the girl, 'I'll love you more if you prove your love for me.' But it's a lie. In Cliff's *Catalogue of the least credible English quotations,* the promise: 'Of course I'll respect you in the morning,' is only *slightly* more believable than: 'The cheque is in the post,' and: 'I'm from the government and I'm here to help you'![3] Emmanuelle-men do *not* respect the women who give in to them; how could they trust them with anyone else? When it comes to settling down, they tend to want a wife who is a virgin. Their view of women is, 'Slightly used—greatly reduced in price.' Instant kicks have long-term kick-backs; and everyone loses out.

Lie no. 2: sex is everything

Emmanuelle tries to make the physical pleasure an end in itself. So the whole point of going out with someone is to spend the night with them after the evening's warm-up. In the words of a song by the late Paddy Roberts it's:

Hiya honey, then hop into bed . . .
to hell with the romance, let's get on with the sex.
© Essex Music 1959

Emmanuelle is taking one aspect of our sexual instinct—the extreme bodily tension and its release—and making it the supreme good. She focuses all the attention and interest on that one moment, and dismisses every other consideration as unimportant. Imagine treating another of our appetites in the same way. Take hunger, for example. It is equally as strong, equally as important and, in many people's opinion, jolly nearly as pleasant! But picture the scene when it is given the Emmanuelle treatment.

A man is sitting in a darkened restaurant. His taste-buds tingle slightly as a waiter approaches with a large, covered serving-dish. Ever so slowly and tantalizingly, the waiter begins to lift and lower the lid, giving momentary glimpses of what's underneath. The customer licks his lips in anticipation. Suddenly, with a magnificent flourish, off comes the lid to reveal in all its glory—a box of Kentucky fried chicken! Saliva trickling down his chin, the man can contain his excitement no longer. He seizes the box and tears off layer after layer of wrapping. At last he holds the coveted chicken-leg; moaning and groaning with delight, he sinks his teeth into the tender flesh and begins to chew. 'Chicken! Oh, chicken!' he sighs, as he savours the succulent taste. But then the taste fades, and all he's got in his mouth is a chewy lump of cud. So he spits it out.

Ridiculous? Of course! He was trying to treat the food as if it only existed for the lovely taste. He was ignoring the fact that food is also for swallowing, digesting and giving you strength. The pleasant taste is an added bonus, but not the whole point of eating.

And Emmanuelle is trying to treat sex as only being there for the lovely feeling. She pretends that it has nothing to do with other levels of togetherness—the companionship of entire lives —mental, emotional, social and economic as well as physical. A cartoon I saw once in a magazine says it all: a man is passionately embracing his 'bunny-girl' (that's right, forget she's a real person) and saying, 'Why talk of love at a moment like this?' And so Emmanuelle cheats you out of 95% of the good that sex is meant to do you. It is a 'fake love', as in the poem at the beginning of this chapter.

And when they're honest, even the Emmanuelle-men will admit to you that it doesn't work. Sex as an end-in-itself ends up just plain boring. Ian Fleming clearly describes himself in his character James Bond, an Emmanuelle-worshipper if ever there was one, in this frank confession that the goddess would rather keep hushed up:

With most women his manner was a mixture of taciturnity and passion. The lengthy approaches to a seduction bored him almost as much as the subsequent mess of disentanglement. He found something grisly in the inevitability of the pattern of each affair. The conventional parabola—sentiment, the touch of the hand, the kiss, the passionate kiss, the feel of the body, bed, then more bed, then less bed, then the boredom, the tears, and the final bitterness —was to him shameful and hypocritical.[4]

Emmanuelle can't deliver the perfect sexual experience. The more you hunt for it, the more it will elude you.

In real life, man (or woman) shall not live by bed alone. There is no such thing as 'casual sex'; it's a contradiction in terms. Sex is part of something much bigger: a personal relationship of loving commitment. Sex and love belong together; sex without love is not worth having.

Lie no. 3: sex is as natural as breathing, eating or drinking

Well, that sentence on its own is true enough. But when Emmanuelle says it, she means you to go on and conclude that sexual activity with whom you like when you like is as necessary, even as unavoidable, as your heartbeat or your next meal. To deny your sexual urges will do you positive damage; probably send you mad or something.

It is here that she falls into her own trap. Sex is *not* exactly parallel to breathing or eating. For one thing, if you don't take a breath in the next minute, or some food in the next month, you'll die. But nobody dies through staying a virgin. In any case, we don't reckon on treating our other instincts to the headlong free-for-all that Emmanuelle wants for sex. People who eat without restraint lose their figure; if they drink alcohol whenever they feel like it, they get a sore head (at the very least!). The good life comes from putting all these things in their proper place. Sometimes saying no not only does no harm, but is also thoroughly necessary and healthy.

Emmanuelle actually wants sex regarded as rather *more* natural than food or drink. She wants it without any limits at all.

Lie no. 4: everybody's doing it

This is a useful one. Nobody likes to feel left out. So if you tell them that everybody else is sleeping with their boyfriend/girlfriend, you should be able to make their reserve and resistance crumble. Boys in particular like to appear to be the irresistible force. You can rely on plenty of them to exaggerate, or even invent, their exploits. Let's face it—if the classroom John Travoltas had actually performed all the heroic feats they say they had, the birthrate would be soaring alarmingly!

Of course, lots of unmarried couples do have sex together, and accept this as a natural part of their lifestyle, whether they're living together or sleeping around. But not everybody! The last thorough survey of the age-range fifteen to nineteen in this country reckoned that 21% of boys and 11% of girls had experienced sexual intercourse. A more recent poll unsurprisingly pushed the figure up to 31%. But it is still not even a majority. So if you like to be with the crowd, *don't* follow Emmanuelle!

Anyway, even if everybody was round the back of the bike shed 'doing it', that wouldn't make it necessarily right. Everybody is selfish a great deal of the time, but it is still better to be unselfish.

Lie no. 5: you're not really a man or woman till you've slept with someone

This is utter rubbish. Seen God's way, the first experience of sexual intercourse is certainly a marvellous moment psychologically in a relationship with someone you're going to spend the rest of your life with. It makes a *married* man or woman of you. But it doesn't make you into a man or woman. Indeed, the reverse because it takes more character, guts and common sense to keep your virginity than to toss it away at the first opportunity—particularly with Emmanuelle's allurements all around.

The full answer to the lie is Jesus himself. He never had sex with anyone, yet he was the most complete, grown-up man who ever lived. He was attractive to women—two of them washed and wiped his bare feet with their hair, and one of them was an ex-prostitute (John 12:1–8; Luke 7:36–50). And he was attracted to women. In an age when they were second-class citizens, he went out of his way to treat them as equals and as individuals precious to God. He moved freely among women, counting many among his followers without the slightest hint of scandal—until *Jesus Christ Superstar* tried to write it into the script and turned Mary Magdalene into his mistress! Emmanuelle is so hard up for convincing evidence that she has to rewrite history to find some.

Lie no. 6: Christianity is anti-sex

Add in a little scare-mongering for good measure. 'Nothing ruins your sexual prospects like becoming a religious maniac. All that praying and fasting and listening to St Paul plays havoc with your hormones. Church folk are all the same, frustrated and repressed.'

I have to admit there is a grain of truth in what she says. The Christian church has a pretty abysmal track record on teaching about sex. One church leader in the third century had himself castrated because he thought that sexual organs were inherently evil and sinful. Another taught that the Holy Spirit leaves the room when a married couple make love. For centuries the church made out that the Old Testament book, Song of Songs, a lusciously erotic love poem, does *not* mean what it says.

But the clue to the whole truth is in that last example. *Christians* may have missed the point completely in times past, and may still have more hang ups than they need have, but the *Bible* isn't anti-sex, nor is Paul, nor is Jesus. They are decidedly in favour of it—at the right time and in the right place.

Here is some advice for husbands:

> So be happy with your wife and find your joy with
> the girl you married—pretty and graceful as a deer.
> Let her charms keep you happy; let her surround
> you with her love (Proverbs 5:18–19).

Or, as the last part is more literally and more red-
bloodedly translated by the New International
Version: 'May her breasts satisfy you always, may
you ever be captivated by her love.'

It's even better in the old Authorized Version,
from a less inhibited century: 'Let her breasts
satisfy thee at all times; and be thou ravished
always with her love.' That doesn't sound anti-sex
to me. It's a positive encouragement to men to
bask in the sexual attraction and attentions of
their wives.

This is what St Paul—the so-called crusty old
bachelor, for ever telling people to stop enjoying
themselves—says:

> Husbands, love your wives just as Christ loved the
> church and gave his life for it. He did this to dedi-
> cate the church to God by his word, after making it
> clean by washing it in water, in order to present the
> church to himself in all its beauty—pure and fault-
> less, without spot or wrinkle or any other imperfec-
> tion. Men ought to love their wives just as they love
> their own bodies. A man who loves his wife loves
> himself. (No one ever hates his own body. Instead,
> he feeds it and takes care of it, just as Christ does the
> church; for we are members of his body.)
> (Ephesians 5:25–30)

This must be the highest recommendation of
physical love in all literature. Sex should be a pattern of Jesus' love for the church and interwoven

with it; it should be as intimate as anyone's care (including Jesus') for his own body.

So to Jesus himself. When he went to a wedding, he put the sparkle back into the party by turning water into wine—600 litres of it (John 2:1–11)! When asked about divorce, he said he was against it because, according to the Maker's instructions, it would spoil and harm sex:

> But in the beginning, at the time of creation, 'God made them male and female,' as the scripture says. 'And for this reason a man will leave his father and mother and unite with his wife, and the two will become one.' So they are no longer two, but one. Man must not separate, then, what God has joined together (Mark 10:6–9).

Jesus and the rest of the Bible talk of God, the Creator who thought up sex in the first place. He knows how it functions best in real life. That's why I listen to Emmanuel and not Emmanuelle. He tells us what sex is really for. He says that marriage is the right time and place for sexual intimacy. Not that everybody in the Bible lived God's way. There are plenty of Emmanuelle-worshippers in its pages, but they're there for us to learn from the sorry mess they got into.

God's point of view raises loads of questions which we shall try not to shirk. After picking holes in Emmanuelle's story, it's only fair to listen to her objections to Emmanuel.

2

Very Good, Says God

The girl entered our hotel room. It was the day after my wife and I had given a lecture at one of the universities in northern Europe. The hotel room was the only place we had for counseling.

She was a beautiful Scandinavian girl. Long blonde hair fell over her shoulders. Gracefully she sat down in the armchair offered to her and looked at us with deep and vivid blue eyes. Her long arms allowed her to fold her hands over her knees. We noticed her fine, slender, fingers, revealing a very tender, precious personality.

As we discussed her problems, we came back again and again to one basic issue which seemed to be the root of all the others. It was the problem which we had least expected when she entered the room: She could not love herself. In fact, she hated herself to such a degree that she was only one step away from putting an end to her life.

To point out to her the apparent gifts she had— her success as a student, the favorable impression she had made upon us by her outward appearance —seemed to be of no avail. She refused to acknowledge anything good about herself. She was afraid that any self-appreciation she might express would mean giving in to the temptation of pride, and to be proud meant to be rejected by God. She had grown up in a tight-laced religious family and had learned that self-depreciation was Christian and self-rejection the only way to find acceptance by God.

We asked her to stand up and take a look in the mirror. She turned her head away. With gentle force I held her head so that she had to look into her own eyes. She cringed as if she were experiencing physical pain.

It look a long time before she was able to whisper (though still unconvinced) the words I asked her to repeat: 'I am a beautiful girl.'[5]

God likes sex. It makes him very pleased. But the tragic thing is that when I say that, some Christians, like the poor girl in the extract above who talked to Walter Trobisch, think I'm being almost blasphemous. They wince at the very sound of the word 'sex'. The church has been influenced for almost all its life by the feeling that, if you can't quite call the invention of sex a mistake on God's part, at least the day he thought it up seems to have been one of his off-days!

For centuries the reaction of the church to sex has looked more like a worried frown than a joyous leap in the air. The impression most people have picked up of the church's teaching on sex is 'Dirty—Dangerous—Don't!'

Two people looking back on the elementary sex education they received at their schools (both with church foundations) describe how it came across to them:

Before we left the Rev. told us not to do it, the doctor told us how not to do it, and the head told us where not to do it.[6]

The timing and the serious atmosphere of this talk left no doubt as to what was really the most important thing in the Christian religion. Since no-one was likely to get married for at least 10 years, the high and heroic task of Christian life was to take the utmost pains (including cold showers) to avoid paying attention to the little devil between one's legs.[7]

Christians always seem to be saying 'No' to it. Whereas God says a loud and enthusiastic 'Yes'. He likes sex. It makes him very pleased. In the first reference to human beings in the Bible—a passage we shall look at in some detail in this chapter—it says, 'God created human beings, making them to be like himself. He created them male and female, blessed them, and said, "Have many children, so that your descendants will live all over the earth and bring it under their control"' (Genesis 1:27–28).

Admittedly, most of us find it hard to work up much enthusiasm about 'male and female' early in life. You're unlikely to have been all that gooey about members of the other sex when you were six. Your attitude was probably more like that of four-year-old Alex who said, 'I want to swop my sister for something better'![8]

Early knowledge about sex usually comes as a bit of a shock. I remember how, when I was nine, I first learned what we used to call 'the facts of life' from a friend at school. I thought, 'Impossible!

27

Men and women clambering over each other? It would be so uncomfortable!' And I firmly told another friend, 'I know that God would think of something better than that!' But hey, am I glad now that he didn't! Because sex is nice. Just think what I might have talked myself out of!

Yes, sex is very nice indeed, even though we first come face to face with it just when everything else in life is topsy-turvy. Suddenly we are at an annoying in-between stage: on the one hand, no longer a child, though parents and teachers often go on treating us as if we were; on the other hand, not allowed to be an adult, free to come and go when we like. We're expected to make all-important decisions about our future, like whether to stay on at school/college or try for a job; but we have no say or vote in how the country's run. We have to live at home still, but want and need the space to work out our own way of doing things. Our families are often infuriatingly slow to understand this! So it's more important than ever to be 'in' with good friends of our own age. The most desperate thing that could happen —and it sometimes does—is to be laughed at or thought odd by them.

So it's not a good moment to have to cope with physical and emotional upheaval as well. But there it is: body-hair starts to grow, girls' breasts develop and the menstrual cycle begins, boys' voices deepen and break. Often the body can't manage all this change without signs of wear and tear. The sheer chemical changes leave many teenagers feeling weepy and depressed without understanding why.

And just when we need the boost of looking good, many of us suffer from our body letting us down again. Our skin goes spotty or blotchy, our hair is lank and greasy, or the growth spurt is all uneven so that the body doesn't seem to hang together properly or be the right shape. A bit like the daughter in N. F. Simpson's hilarious play *One Way Pendulum;* she moodily stares at the mirror and then complains, 'How can I go out with my arms like this? Look at them! . . . They're absolutely ridiculous! . . . If they started lower that would be something . . . Look where they reach to! Just look at that gap!'[9] It's as if we're really seeing ourselves for the first time and not caring too much for the sight.

And that is still not all. *We* may be looking pretty ghastly, but that's when the other sex choose to start looking rather nice. Suddenly girls don't seem soppy any more, nor boys scruffy; they are distinctly desirable. And once again the poor old body doesn't cope too well. *The Secret Diary of Adrian Mole aged 13¾* records typical thrills and spills as the hero, Adrian himself, gets to know his girlfriend, Pandora:

Sunday August 9th
Touched Pandora's bust again. This time I think I felt something soft. My 'thing' keeps growing and shrinking, it seems to have a life of its own. I can't control it.
Monday August 10th
Pandora and I went to the swimming baths this morning. Pandora looked superb in her white string

bikini . . . I didn't trust my thing to behave so I sat in the spectators' gallery and watched Pandora diving off the highest diving board.[10]

Sure; sexual feelings are difficult to control once they take off. But at heart, aren't you glad you've got them? Isn't it a good thing you're not an amoeba whose sex-life only involves splitting in half every now and then?(!) Or a poor old mule, neither definitely male nor female? Or a newt, whose mating pattern is for the male to leave a packet of sperm-seeds hanging on some pond-leaves, for a female to pick up and insert into her own body when he's caught her eye with a court-ship dance?

And isn't it more interesting to be a teenager than a child? Friendship no longer revolves entirely around toys or tennis or stamp-collecting; it takes on a whole new extra world of possibility, of loving and being loved, of attracting and being attracted, of getting a look and a smile and a cuddle from him or her! There's nothing quite like it. An old cartoon in *Punch* showed one girl asking another, 'What's it like being in love, Liza?' 'Coo! It's lovely, Mavis. Like having hot treacle running down your back!'

That's how God has made us to be: 'He created them male and female.' You don't have to pretend that sexual instincts and sexual excitement don't exist. Receive them from God gratefully and enjoy them for what they are. But don't turn them into a god to worship—that's going Emmanuelle's way. Put them into the perspective of four tre-mendously important, encouraging facts that spill

out of these words in Genesis and their imme-
diate setting.

1. Sex is at the heart of what it means to be human

It is virtually the first thing that God is said to
have 'made' us. When you fill in some multiple-
choice quiz or personality test, and they start by
asking your 'Name', 'Age', 'Address', 'Sex'—
they're not nosing into what you get up to in your
spare time; they simply want to know whether you
are male or female, because that is probably the
most vital factor in your character. For example, it
is much more important to who I am that I'm a
bloke than that I'm called Lance, or that I'm
British, or that I live in London, or that I try to
write books for part of my living.

'Sex' here means something much more than
the so-called 'sex organs' in or on your body and
what you do with them. Perhaps it's better to call it
our 'sexuality', because it is referring to what we
are rather than what we do. And our sexuality,
our maleness or femaleness, affects everything
about us. It influences the way we think, the way
we laugh, the way we dress, the way we spend our
time. It colours our moods, our personality, our
opinions and interests, our ambitions and choice
of work. Just imagine how different all these
would be if you were the other sex.

Every relationship or friendship is 'sexual' at
this level, in that our sexuality affects the way we
look at other people—who we like the look of,

and who we are drawn to as ordinary friends, quite apart from special boy/girlfriends.

Love and sex are very closely connected. The warm, happy feelings that good friends inspire in us; the open, trusting sharing—these are part of our sexuality, even when no physical attraction is involved. Self-giving love is the basis of any friendship, and is one of the best things in life.

2. Male and female are different but compatible!

The women's libbers and the unisex brigade have a point. For far too long, men kept all the best jobs and best things in life to themselves. The Sex Discrimination and Equal Opportunity Laws are profoundly just and right in their intentions. God clearly made the two halves of the human race to be equal partners; neither is more 'like himself' than the other.

But when all is said and done, there is still a distinctly marked difference between male and female. Things may no longer be as rigid as seven-year-old Penny wrote: 'Women do the washing up and cleaning and tidying and men go on the train and get tired'![11] But nor are they as ambiguous as six-year-old Paul thought: 'If you put a man and a woman in bed together, one of them will have a baby'![12] There are certain unavoidable physical differences!

There are mental differences too. Men and women think differently, as you can tell from the slightest observation of your parents. In even the most happily united relationship, they have different functions: generally speaking (though of course there are endless variations), he works things out logically, she instinctively knows; he likes to make the final decision, she prefers not to carry the can alone; he usually takes the initiative as the wooer, she is the treasure he seeks.

The way we feel about sex is another crucial area of difference between us. It will be obvious on every page of this book that I am a male of the species. Adult and adolescent males are sexually 'awake' the whole time. Our sexual apparatus hangs outside the body and keeps us constantly aware of our sexuality. There's more than a grain of truth in the standard female reaction, 'You men are all the same; you can only think of one thing!' It's not just 'dirty old men' who have strong sexual appetites and pretty earthy thoughts an inch or two beneath the surface; it is all of us.

For girls, however, the sexual organs are inside the body, and the thoughts are far more tied in with the monthly rhythm. A girl is sexually 'aware', certainly; aware of the boys all round her, and of her effect on them. But she is not instinctively sexually 'awake' in the sense of pining to get physically involved with the nearest available one. But despite the differences, there's a great deal working to pull the two sexes together. Male and female are attracting magnets, not repelling. It's a hopeless task to keep up 'the battle of the sexes', as did the feminist college in Gilbert and Sullivan's *Princess Ida,* with their theme-song:

Man will swear and man will storm—
Man is not at all good form—
Man is of no kind of use—
Man's a donkey—Man's a goose—
Man is coarse and man is plain—
Man is more or less insane—
Man's a ribald—Man's a rake,
Man is Nature's sole mistake.[13]

In spite of all the truth in that, and men's many defects, women still have this delightful habit of falling for us—and we for them. God put it in our genes.

There seems to be a clear order of events in the Genesis description which implies that sexual attraction is more than just the instinct to reproduce and ensure the survival of the race. Undoubtedly sexual intercourse is the way to have babies, and God did say, 'Have many children, so that your descendants will live all over the earth and bring it under your control' (Genesis 1:28) but not until after he created us male and female and blessed us. We *are* before we *do*. In marriage companionship between husband and wife comes before having children. (This emerges more clearly in Genesis 2 which we shall look at in the next chapter.) God planned sex first of all to help us get together.

And so we find in experience. It is almost impossible to put sexual sensations into words, but what we are all aware of, very roughly, is this. An intuitive feeling of wonderful comfort and well-being tingles around what the experts grandiosely call our 'erogenous zones' (lips, breasts, nipples and, primarily, between the legs). This instinctively urges us towards friendship with the other sex in general, and close friendship with one in particular who will match and respond to our sexual 'call'. And from the tremendous surge of fondness and excitement that you release in me when I find you, can blossom a partnership in which you help me to know myself, discover my potential and find out who I really am, and I do the same for you. This process of knowing yourself is the dawn of maturity or adulthood. Our sexuality helps us to grow up.

So every stage of this male-towards-female process is both enjoyable and worth while. Girls mature younger than boys, so there's a spell when same-sex activities are often more popular. But after that mixed schools, youth clubs and holidays come into their own. Mixed activities—games, music, drama, parties, dances; going out together in small groups of two or three of each sex; finding a boy/girlfriend of your own; going steady with one friend for some time; a growing, shared idea that God might want you together for keeps; getting engaged; wedding, honeymoon, setting up home together; facing life's trials and traumas together: babies, unemployment, debt, illness . . . 'for better for worse', but always *together*. That is the general course that God has mapped out for the human race. And he has made us so that, whatever our individual hang-ups and hold-ups, most of it comes to us pretty naturally!

3. Sexuality expresses God's nature

This is difficult for us to wrap our minds round all at once. We're too used to the idea of God being an unsexual 'he'. A little girl called Sylvia once wrote to him, 'Dear God, are boys better than girls. I know you are one, but try to be fair'![14]

But there it stands, inside the one verse: 'So God created human beings, making them to be *like himself*. He created them *male and female*' (Genesis 1:27, my italics). Putting the two thoughts side by side can hardly be an accident. It seems there is a dimension of God-likeness in our sexuality. It is not the only way in which we resemble him—the previous verse, Genesis 1:26, shows that we are also like God in having power and authority over the animals—but 'male and female' is one point of resemblance.

But in what sense can God be said to possess sexuality? Obviously not in the crude, direct sense that he has a wife or girlfriend. But in at least two indirect ways masculinity and femininity have divine origins and can both be seen in God.

First, God's nature has female as well as male characteristics.

'The Lord is a warrior' (Exodus 15:3); 'He is the Lord, strong and mighty, the Lord, victorious in battle' (Psalm 24:8). But he is also a mother: 'I will comfort you in Jerusalem, as a mother comforts her child' (Isaiah 66:13). The most striking expression of this is in the Song of Moses in Deuteronomy 32:18. In its effort to help people understand the poetic language, the Good News

36

Bible hides what is really being said. But the New International Version brings it out clearly: 'You deserted the Rock, who *fathered* you; you forgot the God who gave you birth [*mothered you*]' (my italics).

And when Jesus came to show us what God is like, he naturally had to be born into one sex rather than the other. But he combined a unique blend of male strength with female gentleness. He mastered a donkey-colt that had never been broken in (Mark 11:1–7), but he also shed tears over the fate of Jerusalem (Luke 19:41) with the words, 'How many times have I wanted to put my arms round all your people, just as a hen gathers her chicks under her wings, but you would not let me!' (Luke 13:34).

Even one of the names of God, 'El-Shaddai', usually translated 'Almighty God' (Genesis 17:1), is thought to merge a male name and a female one; El means 'the strong one', and Shaddai perhaps 'the breasted one'. So when God created Eve, he wasn't a man making something different by guess-work, but the male-female Creator expressing the other half of his nature in his human creation.

Secondly, married love of Christian couples reflects the ever-flowing love between Father, Son and Holy Spirit. The picture of God making woman out of one of the man's ribs (Genesis 2:21–22) suggests something incomplete about man or woman on their own. When husband and wife unite, they make each other whole. They light-heartedly refer to each other as 'my other half', or even, if feeling excessively polite, 'my better half'! They establish a small community of warmth and love into which children can safely be born.

Summing up his past ministry on earth as God the Son and his future ministry to his people through the Spirit, Jesus prayed to his Father just before he died, 'I made you known to them, and I will continue to do so, in order that the love you have for me may be in them, and so that I also may be in them' (John 17:26). That the Father's love for Jesus may be in us! What a fantastic idea! And I guess the married love of Christian couples is one of the ways we 'receive' and feel a fraction of the love within the Trinity. In fact, any male-female love can reflect qualities in God's heart that don't come so easily any other way. It is in the nature of love to give generously, to care deeply, to put oneself out sacrificially. Sexual attraction can beautifully heighten the desire to serve and look after the beloved. 'Whoever loves [with the pure, outgoing love that comes from God] is a child of God and knows God' (1 John 4:7).

4. God says sex is very good

He really does (Genesis 1:31)! If you think God thinks sex is naughty or smutty or sniggery, you'd better think again: he likes it! The first thing God tells the brand-new human beings to do is to make love together—repeatedly ('Have many children' [Genesis 1:28])! And this is described as part of his blessing. He could have made the human reproductive system boring or unpleasant, but he chose to combine it with feelings of tenderness, excitement and fun because he loves us. He designed the loving embrace of man and woman —the embrace which ultimately leads to children —as something beautiful, joyful and awe-inspiring. OK, so you may be having difficulty preventing your sexual feelings from sweeping you off course; and people like Emmanuelle distort and pervert them terribly. But God says your sex drives are basically good and healthy and clean— you'd be worse off without them. *He* enjoys them, which means he can help *you* enjoy them and sing a hallelujah chorus about them! He wants sex to be a happy dimension of your life, not a source of worry and fear and guilt. So if you've got problems or doubts or phobias, ask him to sort them out, perhaps even through this book—miracles still happen!

You may be like the girl at the start of the chapter, and indeed like most of us who, when we look in the mirror, sigh, 'Oh dear, we're hardly the approved Hollywood proportions!' But if you dislike yourself and think no one could find you lovable, just you remind yourself that God does. He made you and died for you. If you are a Christian, he lives inside you and has accepted you as one of the family, exactly as you are. Nothing that you are or do can put you out of reach of his love.

And it's not only that he loves your 'soul' in some general way; he loves *you* as the boy or girl that you are, with all your male or female qualities. Your appearance doesn't put him off. He likes your hair, eyes, ears, mouth, nose exactly where they are, because he put them there. They are his handiwork; he thinks they're beautiful.

From the age of twelve till about thirty, I was ashamed of my body. At Christian residential holidays, where I was sharing a bedroom, I didn't dare change or wash in public; I slid in and out of my clothes when no one was watching. All because I once heard my cousin point at a man in swimming-trunks on the seashore and say, 'Yuk! What a skinny man!' I took a squint at the man, and quite irrationally decided that he looked like me. From then on, in my own mind, I was 'Yuk! What a skinny boy!' I had to learn, oh so slowly, that my hands, arms, legs, feet, body didn't worry *God;* he made them! The bits we feel shy or giggly about—breasts, navels, knobbly knees, sex organs—don't embarrass him; though perhaps our embarrassment makes him gently smile. And even if you are going through a clumsy stage of growing at the moment, or if you've let yourself get run down or overweight, spotty or sweaty, he's not going to give up on you. (If it's a real problem, you can always ask a doctor.)

You see, as Jesus, God's been through it too. He had a body very like yours. He felt tired through growing taller; there were days when he must have felt all thumbs; he explored the first prickles of moustache and beard; he felt strong sexual urges and pressures. And he managed it all without putting a foot wrong—morally. The writer to the Hebrews points out that Jesus was 'tempted in every way that we are, but did not sin', so he 'is not one who cannot feel sympathy for our weak-

40

nesses' (Hebrews 4:15). He can help us make good, and make the best of our sexual development.

Furthermore, he shares life with all Christians. Our bodies are his dwelling-place—the whole of them. The Holy Spirit lives just as much in our 'erogenous zones' as he does in our eyes or ears. He can control and bless our sexual feelings and affections as much as our words and worship in a church service.

God says you are a unique, special, beautiful person, including your sexual dreams and longings. Can you, dare you, agree with him and walk into the adventure of loving yourself because he loved you first? It is the first step towards loving your neighbour as yourself, which is part of our high calling as Christians (Mark 12:31); and it is the first step towards being relaxed and confident enough to reach out to be friends with someone else.

3
Marriage

I've got a pal,
   A reg'lar out an' outer,
She's a dear good old gal.
   I'll tell yer all about 'er.
It's many years since fust we met,
   'Er 'air was then as black as jet,
It's whiter now, but she don't fret,
   Not my old gal!

Chorus
We've been together now for forty years,
   An' it don't seem a day too much,
There ain't a lady livin' in the land
   As I'd 'swop' for my dear old Dutch.

I calls 'er Sal,
   'Er proper name is Sairer,
An' yer may find a gal
   As you'd consider fairer.
She ain't a angel—she can start
   A-jawin' till it makes yer smart,
She's just a *woman*, bless 'er 'eart,
   Is my old gal!

Chorus

Sweet fine old gal,
   For worlds I wouldn't lose 'er,
She's a dear good old gal,
   An' that's what made me choose 'er.
She's stuck to me through thick and thin,
   When luck was out, when luck was in,
Ah! wot a wife to me she's been,
   An' wot a *pal!*

Chorus

I sees yer Sal—
   Yer pretty ribbons sportin'!
Many years now, old gal,
   Since them young days of courtin'
I ain't a coward, still I trust
   When we've to part, as part we must,
That Death may come and take me fust
   To wait . . . my pal![15]

Chorus

The second thing God tells us in the Bible about sex, makes it even clearer that he designed it to help us get together. If you ask what sex is *for*, the answer is love and friendship and an end to loneliness.

In Genesis 2, we read of God looking round the Garden of Eden and deciding that there was one thing wrong with it. Even paradise wasn't perfect! 'It is not good,' he said, 'for the man to live alone.' So he resolves to find Adam a partner. 'I will make a suitable companion to help him' (Genesis 2:18). And then, in verses 19–20, comes one of

44

the most humorous parts of the Bible. God pulls Adam's leg by emptying out the zoo he's been working on, and offers him a bride from the birds and the beasts! You can almost hear Adam trying to work it all out. 'Rhinoceros? Shapely nose, but a little on the large side. Hen? Er—does she peck? Porcupine? Ouch—prickly character! Oh dear, are there no other beauties on the short list?'

'Just teasing,' says God. 'I've got a much better idea. Man's best friend won't even be a dog. Look —the missus!' And there she was: Eve—woman, wife, mother. Like the father of the bride, God brings her to him.

It was love at first sight. Adam broke out into the first-ever love song: 'At last, here is one of my own kind—Bone taken from my bone, and flesh from my flesh' (Genesis 2:23). Or as one Irish Bible teacher translated it: 'Whacko, my dear, you're marvellous!' Physically, mentally, emotionally, spiritually, he could tell she was the perfect fit. God had provided him the person to share his sexuality with, in glorious freedom. 'The man and the woman were both naked, but they were not embarrassed' (Genesis 2:25).

That's wonderful enough, but there's even more to it. The mysterious description of God forming the woman out of the man's rib so that the man recognizes her as 'bone from my bone, and flesh from my flesh', pictures a deep truth about marriage. God wants married couples to reach a profound sense of 'we were made for each other'. And they often do. It lies behind the old ideas of marriage being made in heaven, and young men looking for 'Miss Right' to wed.

This experience of belonging and completeness is what marriage is for, even today. God gives us a husband or wife, to rediscover something of the Garden of Eden as we share our lives together. So the Genesis story-teller draws the curtain over their love-making (Genesis 2:24) with words that Jesus echoed and underlined in this way: 'For this reason a man will leave his father and mother and unite with his wife, and the two will become one' (Matthew 19:5–6; Mark 10:6–8).

So when people ask, 'Why are you Christians so against sex outside marriage?', God gives two answers from this Genesis story. The long one is: 'Because sex *in* marriage is too good to miss.' That is why God protects marriage with a high garden wall. On the one side, he uses one of the Ten Commandments to forbid 'adultery'—stealing someone else's husband or wife by having sex with them (Exodus 20:14). Many of Emmanuelle's followers think it's clever, or somehow romantic, to win the affections of someone else's partner. God says it is not clever at all, and brings misery all round. There the joining of bodies, instead of bringing people together, splits them apart. Deceivers and deceived alike all suffer, not to mention the children. God's 'You shall nots' do not deprive us of pleasure; they protect us from pain.

On the other side, God repeatedly outlaws prostitution (Deuteronomy 23:17–18). This is the ultimate form of Emmanuelle-sex, because one person sells their body and time to give someone else a sexual kick, uncomplicated by their not even knowing each other.

But there also seems to be a short answer as to why sex should not happen outside marriage implied in God's teaching. In his sight, sex between two people *is* marriage. When a man unites with his woman, they become one. Sexual intercourse actually makes you married.

Think for a moment what you are saying with your body when you have sex with someone. A handshake is saying, 'Look, I carry no dagger. I trust you. I'm agreeing to dealings with you.' In the same way the 'body-shake' of sex says, 'There is nothing hidden between us; we are completely open to each other. There is nobody else between us; face to face, we are now forming our own new family. We belong to one another so much that our lives have actually entered each other and become entwined. We are no longer two separate people; we are one new unit, part of each other.'

Sexual intercourse is a great deal more than two people enjoying each other's bodies. They are also communicating, speaking to each other in the deepest language there is. Until its purely sexual suggestions took over, 'intercourse' was another word for conversation.

The Bible uses two short, direct words for the sexual act, instead of our rather shy 'sleeping together' or 'making love'. One is 'to lie with', a straightforward description of the physical activity. The other is 'to know', because you never more completely grow in your relationship with your husband or wife than when you lie in their arms and give yourself to them.

Now, how could you honestly say all that with your body while in your mind and under your breath you're contradicting it with, 'It's only for tonight,' or, 'Until her Mum finds out,' or, 'Until I find someone I like better'? You can't say one thing and mean another without it being a lie. And there is no love in that. It is pure (perhaps I should say 'impure') selfishness.

You may like to think you can take someone to your bed to scratch your sexual itch, then toss them aside in the morning like an empty cigarette packet. But that is not the way we are made. The female of the species, in particular, cannot give herself lightly without either being hurt or holding something back.

Arthur Miller expresses well this truth that 'copulation' (the coupling of bodies) actually *means* something, in this snatch of dialogue from his play *The Crucible*:

ELIZABETH: John—grant me this. You have a faulty understanding of young girls. There is a promise made in any bed—

PROCTER: What promise!

ELIZABETH: Spoke or silent, a promise is surely made.[16]

The sheer act of giving yourself is a pledge of personal commitment. If the man then breaks that psychological promise, the woman feels deeply scarred and insulted, wounded and betrayed.

Paul seems to be touching on this in 1 Thessalonians 4:4–6—'Each of you men should know how to live with his wife in a holy and honourable way, not with a lustful desire, like the heathen who do not know God. In this matter, then, no man should do wrong to his fellow-Christian or take advantage of him.' The 'lustful desire', which we shall talk more about in chapter 5, is the plan to have sex with someone who is not your wife—a practice common and acceptable among the 'heathen' or Emmanuelle-worshippers.

To go to bed with someone outside marriage is actually cheating them. It is ripping sex out of its God-given 'home' of marriage and its God-given atmosphere of loving honour. The jewel is no longer in its velvet case, and so you are both deprived of the ecstasy God intends you to grow into in the lifelong commitment and security of marriage. We can only enjoy sexual happiness to the depths that God dreams of, if we know that we belong to each other for ever. Complete abandon is only possible when there is nothing else to worry about. In our sex-life, as much as in every other area of life as a Christian, Father knows best.

The music-hall song that opens this chapter is a celebration of the rich joy and peace of married love. 'Dutch' is slang for 'Duchess'—a lovely compliment to any wife. Share for a moment the excitement felt by some other people who have settled for God's way.

At the lowest level: 'Marriage is popular

because it combines the maximum of temptation with the maximum of opportunity' (George Bernard Shaw). More completely: 'There is no more lovely, friendly and charming relationship, communion or company than a good marriage' (Martin Luther). More mystically: 'It may be conceded to the mathematicians that four is twice two. But two is not twice one; two is two thousand times one. That is why, in spite of a hundred disadvantages, the world will always return to monogamy' (G. K. Chesterton). And more lyrically: 'What greater thing is there for two human souls than to feel that they are joined for life—to strengthen each other in all labour, to rest on each other in all sorrow, to minister to each other in all pain, and to be with each other in silent unspeakable memories?' (George Eliot). Perhaps most fulsomely of all:

> To understand and be understood,
> to know, really know what
> another is thinking,
> to say what you will and
> be sure it is accepted as of value
> or sifted through without reproof
> to be you, really *you*,
> and know you are loved—
> This is near-heaven
>
> (Gloria Okes Perkins).[17]

None of them is saying this to cramp your style or spoil your fun, but simply because marriage is much more fun than just 'living together', let alone just 'sleeping together'. Marriage is true sexual freedom because it sets you free *from* shame, guilt, doubt, competition, fear and a false solemnity in the sexual act itself; and it sets you free *to* concentrate on the needs and happiness of your partner. It combines sex and true love.

Any other sort of so-called 'free love' is a busted flush. It is trying to take shortcuts and ends up being less than human. If it's 'free' in the sense of 'not tied down to one person' then it is not love, because love is commitment through all circumstances. 'Trial marriages' or shacking up with someone 'with no strings attached' are really an insult, rather than a sign of love. They are saying, 'I think I like you enough to commit myself to you, say, 50%; for a couple of months anyway, maybe longer if it works out.' Some basis for unlocking the treasures of your heart!

This is not to say that living together never 'works'. Some couples develop a good relationship and go on to get married. As a Christian, I rejoice at this outcome; not so much because they legalized it in the end, but because they grew into the commitment along the way that turned it from an experiment into a proper, permanent partnership. But it was a stupidly risky way to start. Many other couples (75% of the total)[18] break up after a few weeks or months, with immense pain on both sides, because their relationship hasn't the secure foundation to survive the strains of two selfish people learning to share the same bed and board.

I put it to you. Here are some descriptions of husbands by their wives. Could any of them have reached this degree of affection and intimacy if they were living in an unstable relationship which they both knew could split apart tomorrow if the mood took them?

— A husband is a nuisance I cannot do without!
— To me, a husband is an eternal love affair.
— A husband is someone who surrounds you with such love and trust that you feel free to explore your potential, knowing he will support you, cherish you in your failures and celebrate your success.
— A husband is the man to whom you gave the best years of your life, because he made them the best years of your life.
— A husband is a man who respects you enough to give you his name; who loves you enough to give you his wealth; and who trusts you enough to give you his children.
— Phil is my alter-ego. He is my measuring-stick. If he laughs, I'm being funny. If he understands, I'm communicating and not shouting. He is my father, brother, my best friend, my lover, my critic. All these things I can live without. Why is he so indispensable? Because I'm his alter-ego, measuring-stick, mother, sister, friend, lover and critic. I'm needed.
— He's the guy who makes me say to God every day, 'Thanks for this guy, God.'[19]

The point is that in 'living together' the two people usually remain two through their desire to remain free to pull out. In a successful marriage the two become one, as God planned. They reach a deliciously settled feeling of: 'I just can't imagine —I can't even remember—life without you.'

A husband or wife is the best of God's wedding presents to us. And sexual union with them is another. As divine lover, God showers us with generous gifts. He is exotic in his extravagance. His gifts to us are on an almost absurdly grand scale. For instance, he has made us so that each male 'ejaculation' (the release of seed or sperm that the man plants in the woman at the climax of making love) contains enough cells to produce about 300 million children!

At the same time, as divine artist, God has constructed us with breathtaking economy. Isn't it ingenious and beautiful, for instance, that he combines in that one sexual act the three reasons why he thought up marriage in the first place? Sexual intercourse is the glorious high point of sexual attraction; it is the most intimate way of expressing our longing to care and share as lovers; and it's the way we say, 'Hey! This love is too much for the two of us. We want it to spill over to create new life and have children.'

Christianity went on from this understanding of how God has made us, to one of its most revolutionary social achievements. The ancient world was a man's world. Every man expected to have three women to meet his sexual needs. There was his wife, who would have his kids and keep house; there was his mistress, to be his friend and companion in public; and there was his 'concubine' or prostitute, as his private sex-object.

And the New Testament says, in effect, 'You can scrap that. That's the way to turn women into slaves.' When Paul says, 'Husbands, *love* your wives' (Ephesians 5:25), it is shatteringly new. Because what he means is, 'You should find your lover and sexual partner in one and the same woman—your wife. *She* will be your co-parent, *she* will be your best friend and *she* will be your bed-mate.'

You will never be at peace any other way. God planned sex and marriage to belong together, for our deepest health and happiness as human beings. If you want good sex, you'll have to wait until you get married; if you want a good marriage, save your sex-periments for then. 'Cos that's the way it is.

To which plenty of people shout back, 'Oh no it's not!' I'm no longer thinking of those who recommend arrangements other than lifelong marriage, but rather of those who have suffered the anguish of marital breakdown. How can Christians paint the candy floss picture of marriage that has covered the last few pages when the divorce rate is so high? One third of all marriages in Britain end in divorce. By the end of the 1970s a divorce was taking place, on average, every three minutes. Each year three-quarters of a million people, whether husbands, wives or children, go through the hell of a marriage breaking up. Not to mention the countless others putting up with an unhappy marriage for the sake of appearances or for the sake of the rest of the family. And these sad statistics include plenty of Christians.

Well yes, that's all true. So we'll spend the rest of this chapter trying to work through some of the natural questions about the Christian view of marriage.

1. If marriage is supposed to be so special, why does it go wrong?

There is nothing magical or automatically guaranteed about the institution of marriage. It is simply the vehicle for two responsible, but imperfect, human beings to find their sexual and emotional maturity together. If it fails, one or both of them are to blame, not the marriage-tie. It would be as silly as accusing a car of causing an accident by bad driving.

A teacher once asked his class, 'Now, boys, what is the union of one man with one woman called?' One pupil, searching for the word 'monogamy', blurted out, 'Monotony, Sir'! And indeed, a marriage, like a fire, will go dead and cold if it is not constantly stoked and fuelled.

'The cynic will tell you that married happiness is a matter of give and take,' said Ronald Knox. 'Do not believe him; it is a matter of give and give.'[20] If a marriage is to work, *you* have to work at it. It takes time, effort, humility and (for most people) God's help to learn to care for your partner and be less of a selfish pig. The idle lout who slouches from the pub to his TV armchair, without ever helping his wife, is as surely killing his marriage in cold blood as is the nagging shrew who ceaselessly finds fault with her husband. They are the murderers, not the innocent victims. As Wilbert Gough remarked, 'In marriage, being the right person is as important as finding the right person.' As with all God's most lovely gifts, what is meant to be a foretaste of heaven becomes a living hell if it goes 'off'—like sour cream.

If you know people experiencing marital break-down or breakup, especially the children of such a marriage, treat them very gently and lovingly. It's ghastly. My mother divorced my father soon after I was born. In the remaining thirty-five years of his life he was scarcely ever happy again. Divorce *may* be the less awful of two alternatives. But it is seldom God's way. Even if you ignored him the first time round, he offers to help you say sorry and rebuild what you have broken. For God is in the marriage-repair business.

But for all that, I think a lot of the confusion comes from expecting people who are not Christians, and therefore don't experience God's supernatural help, to live up to Christian ideals. It can't be done. There is a great deal of sense in C. S. Lewis' suggestion:

> My own view is that the Churches should frankly recognise that the majority of the British people are not Christians and, therefore, cannot be expected to live Christian lives. There ought to be two distinct kinds of marriage: one governed by the state with rules enforced on all citizens, the other governed by the Church with rules enforced by her on her own members. The distinction ought to be quite sharp, so that a man knows which couples are married in a Christian sense and which are not.[21]

Presumably such a state marriage would allow the escape route of divorce, and include no vow of 'till death us do part'. Emmanuelle and her agents, of course, go further and positively encourage divorce as an easy way out of any unforeseen difficulties. 'If it doesn't work out, you can always try again.' In 1973 the Divorce Data Company were advertising: 'Our £30 divorce kit includes all forms and complete, easy-to-follow instructions for an undefended divorce action.' It is made to sound so much easier than the bother of trying to save a marriage from ruin.

But Christians would once again learn to regard divorce as the very last resort, because Jesus gives the reason and the resources to keep a marriage alive. Look again at Mark 10:1–12.

2. How do you know the right person to marry?

The one golden rule for a Christian is: marry another Christian (1 Corinthians 7:39). This is not just to be stand-offish and narrow-minded, but to enable you to have a marriage at all. What sort of shared life will it be if you disagree on the most important question: who's in charge? Forget your ideas of, 'After we're married, I'll win him over to believing in Jesus'; he's probably busy thinking, 'Once she's settled down with me, she'll stop this church nonsense.'

Of course, the mere fact that your intended is a fellow-Christian isn't enough on its own. You are looking for a 'suitable companion' for *you*. So it should be someone you respect as a really good friend; someone with qualities you admire; someone you see eye-to-eye with on most things and want to share everything with; someone who excites you and whose company you enjoy. *And* someone you like the look of, sure—but don't make the physical attraction the only or the most important qualification. As Luther bluntly put it, 'Remember, any girl can sleep. Choose one who is some good when she is awake.'[22]

Don't be in too much of a hurry. Drop out of any school-leavers' races to be the first to get married and gain independence (of a sort). Statistically, teenage marriages are three times less likely to last than later ones. Few people at seventeen or eighteen know their own minds as they will in their twenties. Take your time. Look carefully at *her* mum or *his* dad—maybe that's what *they'll* be like in thirty years' time!

Your choice of a marriage partner is the second most important decision you'll ever make, after becoming a Christian. If the devil wasn't able to stop you over that first decision, you can be sure he'll try to put a spanner in the works of this one. So pray regularly for Jesus' help to know whether, when and who. Ask him to give you both a sense of 'rightness'; of 'at last, here is one of my own kind'; of 'we belong to each other'.

My wife and I both had broken engagements to other people before we married each other. In each case, as we stayed open to God's will and leadership, he made it gradually clearer to us that we'd taken a wrong turning. With Sue, there was an 'inner voice' which seemed to say, 'What *are* you doing?' louder and louder from the moment she got engaged. For me, the relationship with my first fiancée grew steadily more difficult, till we had to face facts.

Not that we *recommend* broken engagements—

58

they're painful. It's wisest not to get publicly engaged, nor even 'unofficially', till you can see a definite wedding date at the end of it. Engagement is an unnatural 'in-between' state. You're committed and tied, but you don't yet live in the same house and bed. It's an important run-up to the real thing in which you can double-check whether you are doing the right thing before it's 'too late'. But don't treat it as an emotional stranglehold to hang on to someone you're not really sure about. Better a broken engagement than a broken marriage.

3. Shouldn't we at least try out sex together to make sure we're compatible?

There is a widespread misunderstanding here. Even eleven-year-old Mark had picked it up: 'I shall see how I like being marrid and if I don't like it I will try sumthing else.'[23]

In fact, it is one of Emmanuelle's fabrications to persuade people to shoot the gun. Physical incompatibility is exceedingly rare. Girls' vaginas are almost infinitely flexible; and, whatever they like to imagine, boys' penises, when erect, don't vary all that much in size. The only way anything could go wrong is if one of you is medically abnormal in some way. It's always wise to check with a doctor that you're not, before you get married.

It's Emmanuelle's old mistake of putting the cart before the horse. In this comparison, the horse is your whole relationship, while sexual satisfaction is the cart which follows along behind.

And it will follow smoothly and easily, provided the horse is well fed and happy. Sexual happiness comes when you trust each other and feel secure. You will not trust each other or feel secure if your future marriage is on trial and stands or falls by the sexual thrill barometer. You will have no sexual thrill because you will be uptight. And you may well call the whole thing off, just because you believed one of Emmanuelle's lies.

Learning how to adapt to each other and make your partner sexually happy is all part of the fun and excitement of being married. It helps your love to grow as you share these discoveries together from the start. Don't go picking at the icing before the party—it spoils the cake! The beauty of the honeymoon is lost if you've already tried licking the honey!

4. Why do we have to wait for a wedding? What's so special about the ceremony and the marriage certificate?

Nothing in the Bible suggests that God is all that bothered. What makes you married is the voluntary agreement between both partners that you are moving from being two free agents into one 'spliced' couple; and the consummation of the new relationship when the husband's body penetrates into the wife's. You don't *need* a clergyman or registrar for any of that!

At the same time, Genesis 2:24 links the process of 'becoming one' with 'leaving father and mother'. It is psychologically helpful for all concerned to have some sort of ceremony, however informal, where the parents agree that Bert and Sal are leaving home to set up on their own. It gives the mums a chance to shed a tear or two, and Sal's dad the opportunity to sum things up with a few well-chosen words.

But there is more to it than that. As Christian citizens you have a responsibility to and, I hope, loving care for the rest of your family, your friends, your church and society at large. They all need to know that you are now Mr and Mrs, and no longer Mr and Miss. And they'd like to be there when it happens (well, the ceremony, even if not the consummation)! Is that too much to ask?

You could, of course, write a new wedding service to say: 'We got married in bed last Wednesday night, and these are the promises we physically expressed to each other then.' But I don't think your parents would like it as much as the traditional one!

4

How Far Can We Go?

Boyfriends

To be honest, Lord,
Yes, I do like him.
And he likes me.
He hasn't actually *said* so
But I can tell.
He's really nice, Lord.
You'd like him!
He's kind, and helpful,
And intelligent and sporty,
and good at art—
And simply terrific at the guitar.
In fact you could say
He was re-a--lly dishy, Lord!
What do you say, Lord?
You *do* like him?
Oh great. . . .
But does *he* like You?
Well I don't think
I mentioned that earlier, did I?
No. . . .
One thing he *did* say, I forgot.

No, Lord,
He doesn't like you.
Thank you for reminding me.
Loving You is the most important
Quality that my partner must have.[24]

I'm sorry if the last chapter left you worked up and frustrated. It's easy enough for a happy husband to go on about how lovely it is to be married, and to say that only married people are allowed to sleep together. Obviously that's pretty mean and rough on folk who are not married (yet). Folk, like you perhaps, who are saying, 'What I want to know is, how far can I go with my boy/girlfriend?'

Well OK, let's move away now from the theory to the real questions of how should a Christian bloke and a Christian girl carry on together. What does Emmanuel say about that?

It's going to take some working out. Because there's no such thing as a 'boyfriend' or 'girl-friend', as we understand them, in the Bible. In times when (a) most people married younger; (b) your family often chose who you married; and (c) your time was in no sense your own until you married, the modern boy-girl 'relationship' just didn't happen.

Now of course this does not rule out having a boy/girlfriend. There are plenty of things not mentioned in the Bible—roller-skates, motor-bikes, radio, TV, photocopiers, etc., etc., etc!—which are nonetheless part of God's unfolding plan for the world, and perfectly proper for Christians to have. But at the same time it doesn't

mean we've got a 'no holds barred' free-for-all.
The Bible still says plenty of important things
about relationships in general, in which we must
include the way we treat our boy/girlfriend.

And I think that the first thing we can deduce is
that boy/girlfriends are one of God's loveliest in-
ventions, which he saved up as a bonus for us in
the twentieth century. Often it's not good for a
bloke or girl to 'be alone' in the struggle and pressure of teenage years. And we can find in a steady
friend some of the companionship that God gave
to Adam through Eve. Such a friend can do
worlds of good in keeping us steady at every level
of our lives. Adrian Mole signs off his *Secret Diary*
with the news that Pandora is coming round after
her violin lesson: 'Love is the only thing that keeps
me sane. . . .'[25]

As for me, I'm a pretty shy individual, and so it
took me ages to pluck up courage to ask a girl out
with me. But when I did, and she said yes (!), it
did miracles for my self-confidence. And this love
or friendship, like any close relationship, needs
some form of physical expression. When my
daughter was about eighteen months old, she
sometimes decided life was too much to cope with,
and flung her arms up towards me with the cry,
'Cuggle, cuggle!' She needed to be cuddled and
reassured. In just that way, it can be marvellous to
know there is someone we are special to, who will
care for us and caress us when the going gets
hard, and who we can care for in turn.

But of course the question is, 'Where do you
draw the line between care and caress?' Or, 'When

is a cuggle more than a cuggle?!' The answer involves being open-minded (not making up your own mind too quickly) in several directions all at once.

1. Open yourself up to God

This is the most important section of the whole book. As a Christian, you are not your own boss—you belong to God, and what he says goes. As Paul put it to the Corinthians, when discussing their sexual misdeeds, 'Don't you know that your body is the temple of the Holy Spirit, who lives in you and who was given to you by God? You do not belong to yourselves but to God; he bought you for a price. So use your bodies for God's glory' (1 Corinthians 6:19–20).

God the Father made us. God the Son (Jesus) bought us at the appalling cost of crucifixion and hell in our place. God the Spirit lives in us, and so upgrades our bodies from an animal's trunk into a place of worship. So for Christians, God should have first and last word on how we live.

Which, of course, is very different from how a lot of Christians actually live sexually. Many operate under a sort of 'kiss first, pray later' policy, reckoning that no one's going to cheat them out of their bit of fun, and they'll get straight with God afterwards. You probably noticed how the prayer at the beginning of the chapter started with what *she* wanted, and only gradually came round to what God wanted.

It'll never work. You can't get anywhere as a

Christian, you can't feel God's sunshine on your life, if you're trying to shut him out of one corner. The only way to enjoy life is to keep in step with what God wants. So take it as your number one resolution to make *yourself* happy by making *God* happy. That's how the 'boyfriends' prayer ended: relaxed and grateful in doing God's will. As Paul put it to the Thessalonians, when talking about sexual behaviour, aim to 'please God . . . even more' than you are already (1 Thessalonians 4:1). Never do anything which will make Jesus sad or ashamed to know you.

So, if you're going out with someone, bring God in on the relationship. Don't just go out together, go out together with Jesus. Talk to him together about your love for each other. Any Christian friendship should be making you stronger as a Christian—and a sure test of whether a close friendship is going well is your ability to pray together. This assumes that your boy/girlfriend is a fellow-Christian. This was the issue for the girl in the prayer which opened the chapter. And it's a big issue for many Christian girls.

Largely, I guess, because the Christian good news has been presented in this century in a way that appeals to females—more about the lovely things Jesus will give us than the daring challenge he sets us—the majority of Christians in youth fellowships are girls; and many of us blokes who are Christians seem 'wet' (or at the very least, less macho than our non-Christian contemporaries!). So there's a mighty strong tug on Christian girls to go out with non-Christian boyfriends.

There's certainly no law against going out with non-Christians, nor against being friendly with them. But at the same time, as we've already seen, God wouldn't wish the heartache of a Christian/non-Christian marriage on anyone. So a Christian girl going out *alone* with a non-Christian boy is doing a highly difficult and risky thing. She's got to be ready to make clear from the start that she's a Christian, and to resist his advances if he prefers Emmanuelle's timetable to Emanuel's. And she's got to control her own emotions from getting too involved, by telling herself that this is just a boyfriend and not a potential husband. Some girls cope fine with all of this, but many, if they're honest, know they can't trust themselves. They would do far better to say, 'It must be a Christian boyfriend or none at all.'

And this is where it gets really tough. Because if we mean business in saying, 'God knows best; he tells me what to do,' then we must *all*, boys as well as girls, face up to the possibility that he's going to say, 'No boy/girlfriend at all—at least for the time being.' A special friend is no more an automatic right than a husband or wife. If and when we have one, they come as a precious gift from God. And at the moment, he may be saying to you, 'My way forward for you now is to learn to do without the private leaning-post of a full-time buddy. I want you to discover more of the blessing of having me as your closest friend and support.'

Jesus never asks us to sacrifice our desires for his sake, without making it up to us in a big way. 'Everyone who has left houses or brothers or sisters or father or mother or children or fields [and we could add, 'or boy/girlfriends'] for my sake, will receive a hundred times more and will be given eternal life' (Matthew 19:29). I don't think this means that he's promising a hundred boyfriends later on (either in series, or even more exhausting, in parallel!), but that the lack of one exclusive friend opens us more to the blessing of all our ordinary friends. Jesus is no spoilsport, but always brings us positive good out of what looks like a hardship.

2. Open yourself up to the advantages of having no special boy/girlfriend

To some people, as I've just been saying, this sounds like bad news. But for others it comes as a flood of relief, and for anyone there can be positive value.

A boyfriend or girlfriend is not compulsory! You don't have to have one if you don't want one. Despite every scrap of propaganda Emmanuelle tries to brainwash you with, nobody's a failure or abnormal or immature or repressed or missing out if they go without something they don't really want anyway. If you are happy without a special friend of your own, rejoice! Presumably God wants you without one at the moment, and he's making his will easy for you. There are all sorts of advantages in having no time-and-energy-guzzling relationship going on. God probably wants you to use your time in working, or developing your gifts and interests, in caring for people who need your help or making the most of things you enjoy doing with 'just good friends' of either sex or both. Good friends who share our interests (whether it's shopping or singing or watching football or visiting the housebound) are one of God's richest blessings to us, to be received with thanksgiving.

And if you have a close friend who's the same sex as you, go on—be friends! Don't listen to the Emmanuelle-sneers you hear people whisper, that it shows you must be 'bent'. That's one of her nastiest little distortions. David and Jonathan are the great biblical example of two close friends. David describes Jonathan's love as 'better even than the love of women' (2 Samuel 1:26), because he found Jonathan more of a help and more of a kindred spirit than any of his wives and mistresses. (If he'd narrowed the field down to one wife, he might well have had time to find a love comparable to Jonathan's!) But even the quickest flip through David's love-life reassures you that, as an out-and-out womanizer, he was definitely not bent!

Even if you are unwillingly unattached, try to be positive. If you have just broken up with a boy/girlfriend, allow yourself time to grieve a little. Give the relationship a 'decent burial', sort yourself out, try to think back and learn from it. Why do you feel so cut up? Was it in any way your fault that things didn't work out? What mistakes will you be sure to avoid another time? Allow the Lord to heal any feelings of bitterness you may have towards your former 'steady'. Don't fall straight into the arms of someone else on the rebound, until you are in a fit state to give something good to the relationship.

If you deeply desire a boy/girlfriend, but haven't found one despite many attempts, relax a little. It may be your very intensity that is putting people off. They want this sort of relationship to include some fun, not to be overearnest. Remember that God finds you attractive—you don't have to work up attractiveness on your own. He will make your company more pleasant and desirable to other people as you enjoy his love for you and accept his will for you each day.

3. Open yourself up to the needs of the other people all around you

There is something definitely wrong with your relationship if you and your boy/girlfriend become a 'closed shop'. Don't be an exclusive little huddle so wrapped up in each other that you no longer notice anyone else around you. God still says to you, as to all Christians, 'Love your neighbour as yourself'; and he gives you a close friend to help you obey his commandments, not to skip them. The two of you together can discover exciting new ways to share Jesus' love with others, which you would never have dreamed of on your own.

In particular, alarm-bells start clanging all over the house if you drop out of church, or become useless in your youth fellowship. Time and again one hears, 'We haven't seen Terry for months, since he started going out with Carol,' or, 'It's no good asking Tina to write to visiting speakers any more—she spends all her time with Kevin.'

I know that churches are often largely to blame for the course of true love being a rough ride. Some still seem to disapprove of any romantic attachments in the youth club, and thereby force all friendships into the arms of Emmanuelle. Others are much *too* keen, and exert a terrible pressure for everyone in the YPF to find a partner to pair off with. And almost all churches are gossip clubs where you've only got to show the first glimmerings of interest in a boy or girl for the rest of the membership to start stirring the wedding cake!

This puts immense pressure on us, and we need to do everything we can to help churches be more reasonable. But there is still no excuse for two of us, however much we may be in love, to make other people feel unwanted or shut out of our friendship.

One of the prime ways to do this is to show off physically in public. You may think it incredibly one-up to hold hands the whole way through the mixed Crusader class, and then to have a lovely hug and snog when everyone else has got to make do with a mug of coffee! But if you do, you are causing pain and jealousy, embarrassment and temptation to other people. And Jesus says God really has it in for those who cause upset to others. 'Things that make people fall into sin are bound to happen, but how terrible for the one who makes them happen! It would be better for him if a large millstone were tied round his neck and he were thrown into the sea than for him to cause one of these little ones to sin' (Luke 17:1–2).

4. Open yourself up to your boy/girlfriend

Natural inexperience, together with the ideas Emmanuelle has put around, make us all think, to start with, that a boy or girl of our own is a sort of badge to stick on our front saying, 'Hey, look what a fantastic bird or feller I picked up!'

We begin by looking at them through the golden haze of our own dreams and imaginings. This is it (or rather, him or her)! The boy or girl we've created in our mind with all the desirable features we expect and want in a boy/girlfriend. You know the kind of thing: he/she laughs at my jokes, runs my fan-club, is always there when wanted, licks my wounds, rubs my shoulders. In other words, we start by worshipping a bit of ourselves.

Gradually (or rudely!) we awake to discover that they are real people with hopes and dreams of their own, real fears and problems, real strengths and weaknesses. We learn, often the hard way, the kind of jokes not to crack when they're in a bad mood or feeling down. God has not given them to us as a side-kick to boost our egos but as a Christian friend to help both of us grow up and be built up. He wants *you* to help *her* (or *him*) become more like Jesus. As we get to know them better, we come to realize that they have personal qualities of character—things like

73

courage or cheerfulness or caring—which are a good deal more important than their good looks (or just possibly, lack of them!). Lo and behold, she is not just a lovely bit of fluff, and he is more than a hunk of beefcake!

They're a friend, and friendship is a two-way thing. If I expect her to come along to my cricket match and make the boundary rope look prettier and learn all about no-balls and leg-byes, then she has every right to want me at her sponsored walk, cheering every hundred metres, and paying up with a good grace. We must go to her favourite type of concert as well as mine. Part of friendship is to double the fun of life by sharing, instead of forcing one of you to cut your fun altogether.

Sadly, an awful lot of friendship is bedevilled by selfishness. Like the boy, all gas and no gumption, who wrote to his girl, 'My darling, my darling, I love you, I love you, I love you. I'd come through fire and water to see you. P.S. Meet you Thursday night at the bus-stop, unless it's raining'(!)

Growing *un*selfishness, however, is something that Christians ought to be expert at bringing to their friendships. As we have seen, the Bible certainly recognizes the importance of sexual attraction, but the New Testament never bothers to use the Greek word *eros* (physical love), because it's so excited by an even greater, Christian love. The Greek word here is *agape,* which means putting yourself out to care for someone else. Now, when Christian *agape* enriches natural *eros*, when a boy and girl really care about each other, and live out Jesus' concern for each other, that's worth calling

74

'love'. It's worth bringing other people miles to see and learn from.

One side of the relationship that should flourish in the atmosphere of Jesus' love is respect for each other's feelings. A great deal of pain and heartache in boy/girl relationships comes from not liking or not being able to say what you're really feeling. Many relationships start unequal in the first place. He, for example, just wants an attractive girl to take out and be seen around with, while she is hoping for a replacement for her previously female best friend, someone to talk with for hours about all the new ideas and questions she's thinking through. But neither of them ever says what they want out of the relationship. Neither of them even thinks to ask. Neither helps the other to understand the different ways that boys and girls feel. Both are disappointed, but don't quite like to say so. Consequently, the friendship sputters fitfully for a bit and then sadly fizzles out.

If only they could have learned to talk, to say what was on their minds openly and honestly. But for that they would need to care about each other's feelings, to ask how things were going, to give each other the freedom to voice their doubts and fears, to dare to ask, 'What would you like me to do to make the friendship better?'—and then be ready to do it!

5. Keep your relationship open-ended

One other reason why many boy-girl friendships

go sour is that in the first flush of hope and excitement you never stop to think how it's all going to end. This may sound a ridiculous idea, but it's actually an important piece of common sense, designed to maximize the peace and joy and minimize the pain.

Think about it in cold blood for a moment. Presumably you and your boy/girlfriend don't want to stay as just 'boy and girl' for the next sixty years! In other words, sooner or later (anyway, in the next five years at most), the boy-girl friendship is going to come to an end in one of two ways: either the friendship will get better and better, and at some stage you are going to want to hot it up: first, reaching some private understanding between yourselves, then getting engaged and 'naming the day', then married—'till death us do part'. Or, for one reason or another, you're going to move on in different directions and pull apart and break up. By the law of averages, most boy-girl friendships end this second way. And they usually end in bitterness and accusation as well, because they were not kept sensibly open-ended.

I know a lovely girl who thought she was in the middle of a really happy, exclusive friendship with a good-looking lad. He'd sworn he loved her and that she was the best thing since Princess Diana. And so she was naturally loyal to him— until she came back from a family holiday to find a note out of the blue, saying:

Dear Sandra,
    I've found another girlfriend at home. And as I

don't think it would be right for me to have two
girlfriends at once, I think we shouldn't see each
other again.
　　Yours,
　　Jonathan.

First of all, I felt like kicking Jonathan up the
backside for being so unfeeling towards the girl
whose misery I could see. But then I began to feel
sorry for him, with only Emmanuelle's cruel selfishness to guide him. In the USA they even have
an organization called 'Dumpadate' for getting
rid of unwanted boyfriends or girlfriends! It
sounds quite funny till you think of the human
anguish. That is Emmanuelle at her ugliest, treating people like beer-cans to be disposed of after
use.

When I first started going out with the girl who
is now my wife, almost the first thing I said to her
was, 'For the present we are "just good friends".
*You are free to break it off at any time with no hard
feelings, because we're not deeply committed to each
other.* At the moment we do not own each other, as
if we were married. If either of us wants to move
the relationship up a gear, let's say so—and we'll
talk about it first.' And we did!

In our case, of course, we're still together. But
it's one of my regrets that I cannot still be friends
with a previous girlfriend. Without thinking or
talking about it, we raced ahead emotionally and
expected more support out of the relationship
than we were prepared to put into it. We wanted
each other to be available at all hours, but never
stopped to ask, 'Do we like each other enough, or

have we enough in common, to be this important and this close to each other? Are we really ready to turn the rest of life topsy-turvy for each other?'

We weren't. So when the bust-up came, we had to undo a lot of emotional knots that had been tied too soon. There was anger on both sides. And we have never spoken to each other since. What an unnecessary waste!

Help your friendship to end peacefully by thinking ahead. It's perfectly natural to make plans early on in a steady friendship about how often you want to see each other, and to set a date not too far ahead ('the end of the holidays' or 'Christmas') when you could see whether things are working out well enough to continue.

But here again, make allowances for some very basic psychological differences between boys and girls. From the days of toy prams and dollies, girls are conditioned to look forward eagerly to getting married and having babies of their own. Every boyfriend is met with fairly strong vibrations of 'Are you my future husband?', which immediately puts a bloke into a flat spin. The male instinct is to run a mile from anything which might threaten his independence. And as if she hadn't already got enough grounds to suspect that he doesn't really love her, he is also emotionally able to switch off the relationship when she's not there, and even forget to ring up or write! Don't worry too much, girls—that's just the way we're made. It doesn't necessarily mean we don't love you.

And would you believe it? I've got through five whole sections of this chapter, and I still haven't answered the burning question, 'How far can we go physically?' Typical Christian speaker, trying to chicken out of the real issue! One last chance to redeem myself.

6. Open yourself up to some hard, honest thinking

One of our troubles is that we are inconsistent. We say that we want to be free to work out our own way of living, and that we don't want anyone to tie us down with rules and regulations. And yet, when the Bible gives us exactly that freedom, we blame God for not giving us clear guidelines.

This is the case here. There is *no* helpful chart in the Bible, listing the progression of physical contact:

> Day 1 — hold hands
> Day 2 — kiss
> Day 3 — bear-hug
> Day 4 — deep kissing
> Day 5 — jackpot!

This is because God, in his book, is treating us as grown up enough to work out the right physical expression for our friendship. The only snag is that none of us, not even the golden oldies like me, seem to be that grown up!

And so we need advice. But, please, *advice*—not hard-and-fast rules. What follows is only my suggestion. You are welcome to disagree with it and come up with something better for you— provided you are open to working out what God wants and not just pleasing yourself.

One teenage boy came up with a handy rule of thumb (or of fingers!) which was: 'Anything is allowed so long as it is above the belt.' But that is a rule entirely for male convenience! It kept him from doing anything that would get him into long-term trouble, while allowing him to touch a girl's breasts—to *his* heart's content but to *her* intense frustration.

At the other extreme, I remember hearing a respected Christian youth leader interpret 2 Timothy 2:22 ('Avoid the passions of youth, and strive for righteousness, faith, love and peace, together with those who with a pure heart call out to the Lord for help') as meaning that you should have no physical contact with your boy/girlfriend until you are married.

Wowee! I really take my hat off to him for his extraordinary self-control. And to another Christian leader I admire greatly, who says that the first girl he ever kissed was his fiancée—*after* she had just accepted his proposal! But I simply don't think most of us lesser (or hotter!) mortals can cope with that degree of self-restraint.

And I am quite certain that 2 Timothy 2:22 doesn't require us to. For one thing, despite Emmanuelle's one-track mind, 'the passions of youth' are not *only* sexual. The surrounding verses show that Paul has in mind things like impatience, self-assertion, too quick a tendency to argue, a love of the latest fashion just because it's new, and other strong feelings that young people have, which if uncontrolled would be a disadvantage to Timothy in his role as church leader. But for another, the word 'passions' is a 'thinking' word, meaning 'desires' or 'longings'; it is not a 'doing', 'touching' word at all. It comes in the realm of lust and sexual fantasy, which we shall think about in the next chapter.

The advice I give people when it comes to physical expression is, 'Use your head.' (I don't mean physically, in a sort of friendly head-banging, or a new restriction to showing your emotions only from the neck up!) I mean, *think*! Rumour has it that we all have things called brains up top, and I reckon we should use them to work out our own 'chart' which will pace us in the light of the fact that sexual intercourse *is* marriage.

Now, let's be blunt. You know that I know that you hope this chapter is going to come up with a brand-new revelation from heaven which all the other Christian teachers and sex-books have missed. If only I could announce, 'Yippee, everybody! God's changed his mind. He says that it's OK to sleep with your boy/girlfriend after all.' Actually, there was once a version of the Bible that did say that—by printer's error. They left the word 'not' out of the seventh commandment, so it read: 'Thou *shalt* commit adultery.' It had to be withdrawn mighty fast![26]

God's prescription remains in force: the marriage-act is only for those who are married. This is an extremely helpful guiding principle. If full sexual intercourse is what makes us married, then we can make a firm promise that we shan't do it till we're married. Christian lovers can make a liberating guarantee to each other—which followers of Emmanuelle could never rely on—that neither will push the other to go the whole way sexually unless or until they're married.

This can help us find our own 'sliding scale'. My own view is that on a couple's wedding night, sexual intercourse is the natural progression from the pre-wedding embraces that led up to it. So the appropriate question to ask at every stage of the relationship before that point is, 'How close are we to getting married?' And—crucially important —the appropriate physical endearments should be the milestone at the *end* of each emotional mile, not the sign-post at the *beginning* of it. Too many people think, 'If we push ahead to the next stage of love-making, we shall love each other more,' whereas it works the other way round.

Think for a moment what the various intimacies mean. A simple kiss or an arm round the shoulders are not even exclusively sexual in meaning. Six-year-old Jason got it slightly confused when he wrote, 'Why do all those footballers kiss each other on the telly? They're not married. They're not even engaged.'[27]

I wish in our churches we could all unfreeze and hug each other more, because it's a beautiful way of saying, 'We've sorted out any quarrels we may have had. I care about you and want to help, support and protect you.' That degree of all-round affection, let alone between boyfriend and girlfriend, seems to me thoroughly healthy and desirable. As I once got into the church newspapers for quoting, 'Kissing keeps you slim!'

But that is a whole world away from delibe-rately fondling the sexy parts of someone's body. Can you see that to go that far is to say, 'I have got territorial rights over your sexual feelings. I have permission to work them up when I feel like it'? Now that must belong to a relationship where you are very deeply committed to each other: married, fine; engaged, OK if you know when to stop; 'engaged to be engaged', doubtful—it's so easy to kid yourself that you are in love for ever before you are really sure. The more closely en-twined you are physically, the more agonizing it is to split up.

So if yours is just a good, steady friendship, but not really with marriage in view, even as a distant possibility, then whatever canoodling goes on between you ought, I suggest, to be a million miles short of sexual intercourse. I think, for instance, you'd be mad to undress each other or put your hands under each other's clothes.

Let's be sensible and realistic. A bit of the old slap and tickle, however low-key, is very, very enjoyable. But unless you are strong-willed and strong-minded, the physical side will take over a quite unfair proportion of your time together, and crowd everything else out. I have known young friends of mine take about two and a half hours to 'say goodnight', which does seem a trifle long-winded!

And you know as well as I do that our whole chemistry as human beings makes one thing lead to another. As we get used to kissing *on* the lips, we want to press on to 'French kissing', tongue to tongue inside the mouth. Once we have explored every nook and cranny of someone's body with their clothes on, the pressure mounts to start peeling the clothes off. Naturally, because the whole sequence of heavy petting is heading to its climax in sexual union.

Now, in the end it's up to you to decide where your responsible stopping-places are. I can't do it for you. I'm a fairly controlled customer and can switch off pretty well anywhere at will. But most people find that, unless they're going to inflict great dissatisfaction on themselves, to stimulate each other's 'genitals' (for a boy the penis and testicles, for a girl around the crutch) can only be at most a few weeks away from full bodily intercourse, for many people only a few minutes away. And I am not exaggerating.

There is possible support for all this from a distinctly lurid, '18-certificate' chapter in the Bible, Ezekiel 23. Any deductions from this passage need to be extremely cautious, as it is in picture language. God describes the people of Samaria and Jerusalem as two prostitutes (verse 4), with their willingness to run off and worship other gods as the act of prostitution. In addition, a large part of his quarrel is with their 'adultery', i.e. their taking other god-lovers after he had 'married' them. So there are not many parallels with a twentieth-century boy and girl in each other's arms on a sofa or car back-seat!

But there is at least the suggestion that two of the services illicitly offered by a prostitute are exposing her nakedness, and allowing men to play with her breasts (verses 18, 21). Surely then it is wiser to reserve the stage of love-making where you see and touch your partner's naked body until you are married. A friend of mine offers another piece of advice. He is a bit stricter than I would want to be, but he means it semi-humorously when he says, 'Stay vertical, even when you're engaged; only go horizontal and lie down when you're married!'

Summing it all up, I would give three main suggestions.

1. While I don't understand, and certainly can't in all honesty recommend, a 'general strike' on physical affection, I do advise a 'go-slow'. Go more slowly even than you are already. If in any doubt at all, wait. *If in any doubt at all, wait.* Yes, I did mean to repeat that sentence. It can do no harm to wait, and will probably do good.

I am very glad in my relationship with my wife now, that I never saw a previous girlfriend naked, not even my previous fiancée. That is a memory that can't haunt me. And I don't want it to haunt you either. Don't assume, once you get engaged, that you're 'home and dry'. Engagements do split up, even shortly before the wedding; mine did, and yours might too.

2. *Talk* to each other about what you are doing, even if it's embarrassing to try to find the words to express it. Never feel and caress each other's bodies without discovering whether you are both happy about it. And *never* persist with something one of you is uneasy about. It is unloving and sinful to push beyond what you both feel at peace

with. God can use our consciences in this way to keep our amorous advances in step with his will.

The tragedy of so many relationships is where one partner or both silently believe Emmanuelle's lie that you've got to press on to ever more frenzied heights of sexual gymnastics, even if your conscience is wishing you'd stop. Thousands and thousands of girls have been taken in by the old male trick, 'If you love me, you'll let me.' It is downright selfishness. True love respects and does not force its way. If that boy really loved the girl, he would not try to override her hesitations. It can also be a big help to decide a reasonable limit for your time alone together, and hold each other to it, balancing it with your time spent with other people.

3. If you can't agree, let the girl decide, preferably in advance, where the kissing is going to stop. Constitutionally she finds it easier to put the brakes on early in the process, and is a better judge of when things are in danger of heading out of control. A girl's sexual feelings are like an electric-fire—slow to warm up when first turned on, but burning for a long time afterwards. A boy's sexual feelings, on the other hand, are like a gas-fire—instant ignition, and a pretty quick turn-off too!

5
Learning the Hard Way

In India they tell this legend about the creation of man and woman:

When he had finished creating the man, the Creator realized that he had used up all the concrete elements. There was nothing solid, nothing compact or hard, left over to create the woman.

After thinking for a long time, the Creator took the roundness of the moon,
the flexibility of a clinging vine and the trembling of grass,
the slenderness of a reed and the blossoming of flowers,
the lightness of leaves and the serenity of the rays of sunshine,
the tears of clouds and the instability of the wind,
the fearfulness of a rabbit and the vanity of a peacock,
the softness of a bird's breast and the hardness of a diamond,
the sweetness of honey and the cruelty of a tiger,
the burning of fire and the coldness of snow,
the talkativeness of a magpie and the singing of a nightingale,

the falseness of a crane and the faithfulness of a mother lion.

Mixing all these non-solid elements together, the Creator created the woman and gave her to the man.

After one week, the man came back and said, 'Lord, the creature that you have given to me makes my life unhappy. She talks without ceasing and torments me intolerably so that I have no rest. She insists that I pay attention to her all the time and so my hours are wasted. She cries about every little thing and leads an idle life. I have come to give her back to you, because I can't live with her.'

The Creator said: 'All right.' And he took her back.

After a week had passed, the man came back to the Creator and said: 'Lord, my life is so empty since I gave that creature back to you. I always think of her—how she danced and sang, how she looked at me out of the corner of her eye, how she chatted with me and then snuggled close to me. She was so beautiful to look at and so soft to touch. I like so much to hear her laugh. Please give her back to me.'

The Creator said: 'All right.' And he gave her back.

But three days later, the man came back again and said: 'Lord, I don't know—I just can't explain it, but after all my experience with this creature, I've come to the conclusion that she causes me more trouble than pleasure. I pray thee take her back again! I can't live with her!'

The Creator replied: 'You can't live without her, either!'

And he turned his back to the man and continued his work.

The man said in desperation: 'What shall I do? I can't live with her and I can't live without her!'[28]

On a young people's holiday, my wife and I held a question and answer session about sex. One youngster asked, 'Why is it that our sex-urge can start so early—so long before we can be married? Is God trying to frustrate us?'

It is a question with which I sympathize intensely. It certainly feels cruelly unfair that we become physically capable of reproducing somewhere between twelve and fifteen, but cannot legally get married till sixteen (and, in practice for most of us, much later than that). At first sight, it looks a right mess-up that when our sexual hunger is at its strongest, God says we can't have sex.

But it is not exactly God's fault. It is simply an uncomfortable fact of twentieth-century life—one of the minuses to put against the many pluses of living in a scientifically advanced society. Improved medical and dietary conditions mean that our bodies mature earlier and earlier. But improved educational conditions mean that we reach financial independence later and later. And so the gap of having to wait to get married stretches ever longer.

Most cultures in history, and some in other countries today, have allowed marriage at or before 'puberty' (the physical change from boy into man and girl into woman). In caveman times this physical change needed to happen fairly early if the race was to survive in a dangerous, untamed world. But now that life for most people is so much safer, and yet so much more complex, our culture doesn't encourage marriage till at least three or four years after puberty. You may be old enough to conceive a child, but are you equipped to provide for it yet?

Life in the waiting period is undoubtedly hard, but let's try to look at it positively. The teenage years are God's 'L-plates' phase. In every area of life we are learning, training and gaining new experience to equip us to be adults. No worthwhile skill is ever acquired without time, patience, dedication and hard work. Even if you had it in you to be a great sportsman, you couldn't be a champion tomorrow. That degree of self-mastery takes months, even years.

And it is just the same with our sexual development. As sex is probably the hardest (and most rewarding) area of life to master, it's a challenge worth rising to. You couldn't be a good spouse or parent tomorrow, but there's every chance you will be good in time, if you use your opportunities well now. Your teens are the time to pick up the secrets that will lead to a happy sex-life: learn how to control your sex-drives, rather than let them control you; discover how the other sex ticks, and what qualities you admire and would like to live with in a future marriage partner; practise the skill of being a faithful friend who works at a relationship through bad times as well as good; develop into a less childish, selfish person. In this way you go through, and pass beyond, the process described in the Indian legend with which the chapter began.

All teenage experience, provided you learn from it, goes into the bank to help you become a better lover, carer, husband/wife, father/mother, when the time comes. And you can forget the idea that you're a victim of a double standard which requires teenagers to grit their teeth and practise relentless self-control, while married adults let themselves rip in a wild orgy of permissiveness! Most married couples can't and don't make love every time either partner feels like it—they'd never get anything else done! The Christian way is to put your partner's sexual needs first, and learn self-control. 1 Corinthians 7:3–5 drives selfishness out of the marriage-bed.

For a human being, and especially for a Christian, self-control in one form or another is a permanent calling. The alcoholic or compulsive gambler, the person who has never learned to bridle his temper or tongue, all are walking disaster-areas who wreck their own lives as well as threatening untold damage to others.

No wonder the Bible writes self-control into the program for every Christian. The lack of it is a killer (Proverbs 5:23). The possibility of achieving it is part of the Christian good news (Acts 24:25). It is an attractive quality, one part of the 'fruit' that the Holy Spirit comes into our lives to produce (Galatians 5:22–23; 2 Timothy 1:7). It must be at the heart of Christian family and community life if they are to sparkle with God's beauty in an ugly, godless world (Titus 2:1–12).

The battle for self-control is won or lost in the mind. Our thoughts and attitudes dictate what we do. And nowhere is the fight for sexual self-control and purity more obvious than in our thoughts. Let's take a couple of examples of imaginary but typical people, borrowed from one of the Serendipity Youth Bible Study books, to illustrate some of the ways God helps us to fight and win the battle of the mind.

Case history 1: Joanna

Jo wasn't a Christian at school. She was a very attractive girl, fun to be with, and enjoyed the attention of boys, the closer the better! She could play hard to get, or give boys the come-on, depending on her mood or feelings at the time. She knew how to dress to attract their attention, yet still be accepted by the other girls. By the time she was 17, she made out that she had lost count of the boys she had slept with, and had no intention of giving any of that up.

So when she became a Christian in her late teens, she reckoned it was her inner attitude to Jesus that was important, not all the do's and don't's. 'Love' was the great principle, and 'making love' was surely just part of that. She thought that she could be a witness for Jesus to the current boyfriend in the back of a car or van as easily as anywhere else.

But to her surprise she found her attitude changing. It was not an instant miracle, but the process of God gradually changing her mind and heart from the inside out. One thought, one opinion, one action at a time. Over many months she began to feel bad about treating sex so lightly; she wanted to make a fresh start and to keep herself for 'the right one'. But perhaps it was too late. . . .

Case history 2: Joseph

Joe's early experience of sex was pretty normal: an undressing session with his girl cousin when they were both seven!

He only got really interested when he started doing a paper-round in the third year at school. He stopped off on the way to have a good look at page 3. And then the shop-owner began giving him back numbers of 'Men Only'! He drooled over the pictures and read the stories again and again, imagining himself as the dashing lover. Every girl he saw, he visualised as one of the pin-ups from the magazine: undressed and outrageously over-endowed!

The trouble was, as time went on, 'Men Only' seemed a bit tame, so that he started ferreting for something more pornographic; and instead of feeling more at home with girls, he grew more shy of them and less able to build a relationship with a girlfriend of his own.

One night he plucked up courage to talk to the leader of his youth fellowship, who helped him to see that although the magazines made him *feel* sexually expert and grown up (temporarily), they were actually preventing him from growing up in real life.[29]

What the Jo(e)s need to know

1. Guilt and forgiveness

A sense of guilt or shame is one of the chief obstacles to sexual happiness. The basic awareness of what is right or wrong is set by God, and helps to guard our sexuality for the life-enriching uses he has in mind. Many people feel guilty because they have misused sex in one way or another.

Our conscience is like a moral compass-needle pointing towards God's true north. But because of 'enemy interference', it is not wholly reliable. Sometimes it is under-active, as with Jo before she became a Christian. Sometimes it can become over-active, as it had by the time she feared she had done too much wrong to be allowed a fresh start.

A guilty conscience may well be the Holy Spirit trying us and convicting us in God's court. He is urging us to see the error of our ways and to mend them. This was the case with Jo as she began to realize that it was not on as a Christian to give her body to a series of boys, while saving the rest of herself for a future husband. With her, guilty conscience reflected real guilt.

But equally, a guilty conscience can be the product of false accusations from Emmanuelle's boss, the devil, whom Jesus called 'the father of lies' (John 8:44). One of his lying accusations, which many people struggle under, is that sexual sins are worse than other sins. They are not. They may be vivid and stick in our minds, but God does not rub our noses in them. Jesus was compassionate towards the prostitutes, who knew their own wretchedness and wanted release from a system in which they were as much victims as villains. But he was flint-hard against the chief priests and elders who hypocritically prided themselves on their outward virtue, but refused to help the down-trodden (Matthew 21:28–32). We would do well to check our scale of values by his.

One area of widespread false guilt is the one that trapped Joe—'impure thoughts'. Ironically, one of Jesus' own teachings has contributed to over-burdened consciences, because Christian teachers have been pretty merciless in how they have explained it. In the sermon on the mount,

Jesus said, 'You have heard that it was said, "You shall not commit adultery." But I say to you that every one who looks at a woman lustfully has already committed adultery with her in his heart' (Matthew 5:27–28, RSV). From this, every knowing chuckle, every wolf-whistle, every sexual fantasy has been branded as sinful lechery.

We need to think a bit more clearly about what Jesus was saying. His point in Matthew 5 is that the Old Testament law is a lot more demanding than the 'technical' obedience that the Pharisees gave it. It is possible to break God's commandment in your mind, while apparently obeying it on the surface. As with adultery, you may never actually have nicked your neighbour's wife, but God says it is as bad in his sight to have thought of doing so.

The word translated 'lustfully' is the same as 'passion' in the last chapter. It means 'to set one's heart on', 'to desire strongly'. The Good News Bible gives a helpful, if rather cool, translation of verse 28: 'Anyone who looks at a woman and wants to possess her.' It's more than just wanting to; it's relishing the thought. In other words, it is deliberately looking at a particular woman (or man) as a sex-object.

King David committed adultery with Bath-sheba. The idea came to him one afternoon as he sauntered on the palace roof, and saw her taking a bath. He found out who she was and sent messengers to fetch her (2 Samuel 11:2–4). What Jesus is saying is that David would still have been guilty of mental adultery, even if she had said no and jumped off the roof.

So, have you sinned against Matthew 5:28? Well, not by what we all do when we arrive at some inter-school event, or Christian holiday, or maybe when we leave home for the first time— 'surveying the talent' and dividing it up into the pretty, the ugly and the pretty ugly! Nor by thinking, 'Cor, what a smasher!' Nor necessarily by that natural question which pops into our minds, 'I wonder what he/she looks like with no clothes on.' Nor even by the very understandable guessing and imagining what sexual intercourse must feel like (without anyone particular in mind). This is all normal, healthy sexuality.

But as the old saying goes, although you can't help birds flying over your head, you can stop them building nests in your hair! Each of these natural sexual reactions can become lust if you let it stick around for too long. For lust is, as Jesus puts it, committing adultery in your 'heart' or imagination. It is stripping and having sex with someone in your mind, whether it is a real 'playmate' whom you know, or some photo of a girl in a magazine.

So the important thing is not to let the first look become a second-look-for-the-wrong-reason! Let Jesus in on how you feel. 'She's beautiful, isn't she, Lord?' is a great way to stop your thoughts going sour, turning the natural enjoyment of a lovely creature into praise of the loving Creator.

This is the ideal to aim at, and keep aiming at. But it is undeniable that we all fail, frequently. And if, like Joe, you really have given in to

impure thoughts or any other sexual wrongdoing
—and who in their teens has not?—come and sort
it out with Jesus. He knows what you've done. He
understands. And he's longing to put you right
again. Don't think it's unforgivable. He can certainly wash you clean and give you a new start,
because on the cross he died for your sexual sins
as much as for any others.

Just listen to some of God's promises of forgiveness, and let them do you good.

The Lord says, 'Now, let's settle the matter. You are
stained red with sin, but I will wash you as clean as
snow. Although your stains are deep red, you will be
as white as wool' (Isaiah 1:18).
I will sprinkle clean water on you and make you
clean from all your idols and everything else that has
defiled you (Ezekiel 36:25).

And another prophet praises God for his forgiveness in these terms:

You will be merciful to us once again. You will
trample our sins underfoot and send them to the
bottom of the sea! (Micah 7:19).

All that God asks us is to 'confess' our sins to him
(1 John 1:9). This means to own up that we have
done wrong; to agree with him that we have
broken his law and displeased him; to admit that
it's our fault, without trying to wriggle out and
blame someone else. Then he keeps his side of the
bargain; he forgives us and purifies us. In his
sight, it's just as if we'd never sinned at all.

2. *Strength and weakness*

The good news isn't only that God forgives what we've done wrong. He also brings strength to do right in the future. When they brought him a woman caught in the very act of having sex with someone not her husband, Jesus said, 'I do not condemn you. . . . Go, but do not sin again' (John 8:11). In other words, 'I can and will forgive your sin. But don't think that means it doesn't matter; it is still sin. I want you to learn to live free from that sin.'

That woman was morally weak, and so are we. We all find sexual temptation almost impossible to resist on our own. It is most unlikely that, in her case, 'getting off with a caution' would have been enough to keep her on the straight and narrow from then on. Jesus' words would only have been permanent good news to her, if she could receive some inner strength to reinforce her conscience and her will against her uncontrolled instincts.

And that is exactly what Jesus offers to every Christian. For all of us it is true that 'God is always at work in you to make you willing and able to obey his own purpose' (Philippians 2:13). I love that '*willing* and able'. He not only gives us the strength to follow his will; he changes our desires to *want* to, as well. This is what Jo found happening, as her determination to go on enjoying sex outside marriage began to fade away. Sometimes if we are very attached to a wrong practice or train of thought, we need to start by praying, 'Lord, make me willing to be made willing to see it your way!'

When we are open to God, he can shape us up to live his way. Jesus 'can help those who are tempted, because he himself was tempted and suffered' (Hebrews 2:18). He doesn't cushion us from the battle, any more than he cushioned himself. He leaves us in the thick of the fight, which he also had to fight; but he joins us and strengthens us by training us to rely on his strength. It is not a 'shall-I, shan't-I?' struggle on our own, which we would lose every time, but a resolute defence and attack with Jesus' weapons.

When I became a Christian in my teens, the temptation to think impure thoughts was never far away. I remember having to learn almost at once to get used to talking to Jesus in prayer at every spare moment, so that it was natural to call on him in the emergency. The growing awareness of his presence with me was a powerful tonic. When I felt myself slipping, I could reach out for his grasp with the words, 'Lord, hold me and help me.'

And I found it helpful to learn verses of the Bible to quote at the devil or at myself, as Jesus did when tempted. The dagger I used again and again to point at the enemy was, 'Go away, Satan! The scripture says, "Worship the Lord your God and serve only him!"' (Matthew 4:10). And, when I needed to give myself a talking-to, the shield I sheltered behind was, 'God keeps his promise, and he will not allow you to be tested beyond your power to remain firm; at the time you are put to the test, he will give *you* [Lance Pierson], the strength to endure it, and so provide you with a way out' (1 Corinthians 10:13, italics mine).

In all of this, our overall motive is critically important. As we have seen, Paul's general sex education for the Thessalonians was to 'live in order to please God' more and more (1 Thessalonians 4:1). His encouragement to assure them that it would be possible was the reminder that God 'gives you his Holy Spirit' (1 Thessalonians 4:8). The very Father God, whom we're trying to learn to please, is right there with us, *inside* us! He is there to show us what will make him happy and how to do it.

Both Jo and Joe needed to work out more of what it means to please God and to follow the Holy Spirit's guidance, in the way they explored and expressed their sexuality. Here are some examples of how I think it might pan out for us.

1. Dress

By all means dress fashionably and colourfully in clothes that are 'you'; but not deliberately to turn other people on. That's doing Emmanuelle's work for her. Girls don't always realize how see-through or skin-tight clothes can turn us poor weak males to jelly! Let the Holy Spirit guide your shopping.

And at least listen to his scale of priorities, put on record in Peter's first letter:

> You should not use outward aids to make yourselves beautiful, such as the way you do your hair, or the jewellery you put on, or the dresses you wear. In-

stead, your beauty should consist of your true inner self, the ageless beauty of a gentle and quiet spirit, which is of the greatest value in God's sight' (1 Peter 3:3–4).

Peter's point here is not that we should set out to be plain and dowdy, but that beauty of character is even more important than beautiful looks. And the fact that he happens to be talking to Christian wives of non-Christian husbands doesn't necessarily make this a girls-only instruction. If only Christian blokes would *pray* as often as they *spray* sweet-smelling aerosols!

2. Pictures

How the explicit bits of general release films influence you depends on your own threshold. You need to ask God to show you where you are in danger of stumbling over into displeasing him. By and large, girls are less affected by what they see than boys are. But even among blokes there are wide differences. I'm hopeless—the slightest hint of 'four bare legs in a bed' is enough to work me up, but I know people who tell me they've watched the most torrid love-scenes without turning a hair. Well, bully for them; they find films less of a mine-field than I do.

But I wouldn't under any circumstances recommend what the posters misleadingly call 'adult films' or the videos in sex shops. It's not really adults who go to see them; it's sad people who have got stuck in their development and aren't able to achieve a happy sex-life with a wife or husband. They feel the need to get their kicks by watching other people. God understands their plight but he can't be pleased with it, because it has removed sexual arousal from a loving personal relationship, which is where he planted it.

Much the same goes for pornographic magazines, as Joe came to understand. *Playboy* and *Playgirl* are quite well named; they are for people who are still children sexually, wanting to play around instead of growing up and living in the real world. 'Haven't you learned to make friends with real people yet?' is quite a good put-down to the guys who think it looks big to pass naughty photos along the back row in class—provided you can say it with a smile, and without sounding prudish.

3. Jokes

You may feel that God would never be pleased with a sex joke, and that you should never pass one on. I respect that point of view, but personally feel that trying to please God doesn't mean we have to give people the impression that we are 'holier-than-thou' freaks. For years I was a terrible hypocrite. Although my mind was like a sexual cesspool inside, I thought I had to be all disapproving on the outside.

So when friends at school told sex jokes, I looked down my nose and never smiled. I suppose if they'd asked why, I'd have said, 'You shouldn't make fun of something meant to be sacred.' It took me years to see that as well as being a beautiful gift from God, sex *is* fun, and therefore often funny. Of course, some sex jokes are revolting and leave you feeling sick or dirty—forget those. The Bible says, 'Nor is it fitting for you to use language which is obscene, profane or vulgar' (Ephesians 5:4). But some sex jokes are not obscene (i.e. repulsive, loathsome, grossly indecent), they are just plain comic—so why not laugh?

I think that part of the reason why the Song of Songs is in the Bible is to illustrate both the beauty and fun of sex. As well as being a series of beautiful love poems, parts of it are deliberately funny —and yet they manage to be explicit and clean and healthy at the same time. What interests me is that they are far more liberated than much of our so-called 'permissive', Emmanuelle-minded twentieth-century manages to be.

One year I kept the Valentine cards my wife and I sent to each other. One is a typically male offering, featuring a boy-mouse in a blue bow-tie, saying: (page 1) 'You set my heart on fire!', (page 2) 'and I'm burning with DESIRE!' Her card to me showed two small puppies, one of them with a pink bow-tie (!), whispering: (page 1) 'Psst . . . Valentine, I'm the *reserved* type. . .', (page 2)'. . . reserved for *you*!' Is that really the best we can do to say, 'I love you'? Do we have to use fluffy little animals to carry our messages for us?

Solomon can teach us a thing or two. He was what you might politely call a naughty boy. He had not just one wife, but 700 of them—and 300 mistresses waiting in an antechamber, for when he got tired of the legalized lot! I reckon that leaves Emmanuelle toddling in the nursery class!

And if you're puzzled at what such a sexual superstar is doing in the Bible, bear two things in mind. One is that it was the custom for kings in the ancient world to demonstrate their power and prowess by marrying (and thus owning) as many foreign princesses as possible; and their wealth by maintaining the largest colony of concubines (or 'bits on the side') that they could afford. The second thing to remember is that while the Bible *records* Solomon's marital statistics, it does not *recommend* them. Indeed, it blames them for his sin and disgrace (1 Kings 11:1–6). The Bible contains many characters who go against God's plan. But while condemning them, it does not lose sight of what is human, and in this case humorous, about them.

In this part of one of Solomon's songs (Song of Songs 4:1–6), we eavesdrop on him chatting up the latest recruit to his harem. Imagine wooing your girlfriend like this:

How beautiful you are, my love!
How your eyes shine with love behind your veil.
Your hair dances, like a flock of goats
    bounding down the hills of Gilead.
[Thinks: some hair conditioner!]
Your teeth are as white as sheep
    that have just been shorn and washed.
[Good toothpaste too.]
Not one of them is missing; [*and* a good dentist!]
    they are all perfectly matched.
Your lips are like a scarlet ribbon; [Bright lipstick]

104

how lovely they are when you speak.
Your cheeks glow behind your veil.
Your neck is like the tower of David,
  round and smooth,
  with a necklace like a thousand shields hung
  round it.
  [Every seducer enjoys a challenge.]
Your breasts are like gazelles,
  twin deer feeding among lilies.
  [Go on, I dare you to tell your girlfriend that!]
I will stay on the hill of myrrh,
  the hill of incense
  [She'd obviously got some most superior
  perfume],
  until the morning breezes blow and the darkness
  disappears.

What a perfect description of making love! And
that's the Bible!

Christians are just as keen to uphold the sixth
commandment, 'Do not commit murder,' as they
are the seventh, 'Do not commit adultery.' They
should therefore dislike wallowing in unnecessary
displays of violence. And yet they are able to dis-
tinguish between 'the real thing' (video nasties)
and the stylized cartoon joke (Tom and Jerry)
which is funny. But at the same time, we seem
unable to see the difference between pornography (literally, descriptions of prostitution, and
so any form of material deliberately exciting you
to want Emmanuelle-sex), and a harmless recog-
nition that the sexual side of life doesn't have to
be desperately serious the whole time.

4. Information

And of course, learning to please Jesus in the way that we live doesn't mean that we have to shut our eyes and stay absolutely pig-ignorant about everything to do with sex. There is quite enough ignorance around already. In one survey of teenagers, when asked the question, 'Are you a virgin?' a girl replied, 'Not yet'; and an intelligent boy replied to the question, 'What do you know about V.D.?' with, 'Nothing, unless you mean Vapour Density.' In these areas to know nothing can be not only embarrassing but dangerous. God would be more pleased for us to know. We all have many questions and problems. And it's quite OK to find out the answers—as long as we're aiming at Emmanuel-sex, not Emmanuelle.

The question is, where to ask? You can start by reading some helpful books (I list a few at the back of this book). And it would also be good, wouldn't it, to find someone you trust (maybe a close friend, or a sympathetic Christian adult, as in Joe's case) to talk about whatever's on your mind. If there's absolutely no one in your neck of the woods, you're welcome to try writing to me (c/o Kingsway Publications). In any case, it's sometimes easier to talk to a stranger without having to look him in the eye.

From there perhaps we can move on to some realistic, down-to-earth discussion in Christian Unions and youth groups, to work out together how we can help each other in this high and mighty task of pleasing God.

But remember that some people find sex difficult to talk about, and nobody should be forced to against their will. In fact, it's often parents or youth leaders who find it hardest to talk about sex. One generation has a natural shyness and uncertainty in discussing personal matters with another. We're not sure how much 'they' really know.

Like the small kid who asked his mother, 'Mum, how was I born?' And she said, 'Well, dear, we found you under a gooseberry bush.' He looked a bit puzzled at this. 'Oh! Well, how were you born, Mum?' This time she tried, 'Er—the stork brought me to your granny.' 'Oh!' he said, still more uncertain. 'Well, how was Granny born, then?' Mum was scratching her head by now, but she came up with, 'Your granny started life as a twinkle in your great-grandad's eye.' This at last was too much for the young chap, who exploded, 'I'm really worried about our family. We haven't had a normal birth in three generations!'

Six-year-old Vivienne makes a perceptive point about family inhibitions that we might do well to overcome: 'When you are a baby you can see your mummys bosum but when you grow up its not alowed and I think thats a silly rule.'[30]

Thoughts, fantasies, clothes, films, books, jokes, questions, problems, someone to talk to—there's no easy answer to any of these. We have to learn the hard way. But at least we can learn and grow, steadily, surely, as the Jo(e)s did. And with Father God there to trust and to please, Christians can rest assured that we won't lose out.

6

Just Me and Myself

I have to do it.
I can't help it, Lord.
The pressure builds up
deep inside of me
until there is no relief.
I have to do it.

It's like a deep thirst,
the kind that reaches
far beyond the throat.
I can last just so long
and then I can't stand it anymore.
I have to do it.
At least that's how I feel.

No one talks about it much.
But most of the kids
do what I do.
Some don't admit it
and others laugh about it.
But I don't understand
why we can't find a way
to be honest and open about it.

My parents and teachers
tell us to play sports,
or read a good book,
or go out with friends,
or pray about it.

But that doesn't solve it.
When I'm alone
the faces and bodies
of people I know
flash into my mind
and I can't help
thinking about it.

It's part of me—
a good part of me, I hope.
But I get the impression
from adults I know
that I'm rather weak
or disturbed
or sick
or something
if I can't suppress
these thoughts and feelings.

When I try to fight it
I feel as if I could explode inside
and I want release
more than ever.

I enjoy other kids.
I enjoy school.
I enjoy sports.
I enjoy being alive
with adults and friends.

But all of this contact
only seems to intensify
that deep thirst
to touch my body
and love myself,
when I'm alone.

I imagine myself alone
with one of the kids I like.
I remember the eyes,
the laugh,
the smooth hair,
the cheeks,
the warm skin
and I want them
close beside me.

But something is wrong.
It eats away at me
until I feel miserable
and very very lonely.

What I want is a way
to face these feelings,
to understand myself,
to be proud of myself,
to build myself,
and to be myself
without hurting myself.

Lord,
give me someone
who is honest enough
to admit these desires,
and to help me grow
without pretending

that God or good people
have an easy answer for me.[31]

'It's part of me—a good part of me, I hope. . . .
But something is wrong.' For many, many years
my most pressing sexual problem was 'that deep
thirst to touch my body and love myself'. It is
technically known as 'masturbation', and many
people find it a highly embarrassing subject. Some
would genuinely prefer not to discuss it at all;
others are just confused by this long, medical-
sounding word—'mass-der-whatsit?'

It may be, particularly if you are a girl, that it
doesn't interest or affect you at all. If so, do feel
free to give this rather personal chapter a miss. I
promise I shan't be offended!

Twenty years ago the Schofield Report *The
Sexual Behaviour of Young People* was published. It
was based on 2000 interviews with people
between the ages of thirteen and nineteen. At the
end of the interview they held a talk-back on questions that had been difficult to answer or understand. On the subject of masturbation, one boy
said, 'It's all right to ask, but change the word.'[32]

I agree—it's an ugly mouthful. And the word
they write on the walls of public conveniences—
'wanking'—is hardly any more beautiful. Masturbation simply means playing with yourself. Or, to
be more precise, a boy rubbing his penis, or a girl
her clitoris, till they reach a sexual climax. So for
the rest of this chapter, I shall call it instead 'sex
by yourself'.

During my first seven years as a Christian, I

heard quite a number of pep talks about sex. But none of them ever mentioned sex by yourself. And as I heard these speakers wandering round the subject with words like, 'Marriage—marvellous, marvellous! And girlfriends—well, yes if you must! But impure thoughts—tut, tut, tut! OK, then, folks—that's all,' I formed two clear ideas.

One was that obviously the thought of sex by themselves had never even occurred to them, and that I was the only person having difficulty. And the other was that perhaps sex by yourself was *so* dreadful that it was unmentionable! Either way I was trapped. I built up a whole load of guilt for the fact that from my mid-teens till I got married, I had sex by myself two or three times a week, sometimes more.

I hated myself for it. I prayed unsuccessfully for deliverance. I wrote an anonymous, typed letter to the publisher of a forthcoming book of answers to sexual problems, saying that my experience felt just like James 1:14–15: 'A person is tempted when he is drawn away and trapped by his own evil desire. Then his evil desire conceives and gives birth to sin; and sin, when it is full-grown, gives birth to death.' Sadly, the book was never published, so I didn't get my answer!

I had to try my own remedies. I made myself go jogging to 'mortify the flesh'. And I used to punish myself by going without chocolate and paying money to charity—twenty-five pence each time! And that was a lot of money in those days! I even wrote a letter to myself, which I still have, saying, 'You are jeopardizing seriously your chances of ever reaching those pearly gates' (posh, eighteen-year-old language for 'you'll never get to heaven, mate'). I could not see how God could possibly forgive me so many times. Surely he would have to send me to hell. In other words, the devil had got me exactly where he wanted me—under his thumb—and was saying, 'You've really gone and done it now, you maggot!'

When I turned to Christian books, I did not find much comfort. Even the two that were the most helpful on general questions let me down with a bump. For although both said you needn't get too worried about sex by yourself, neither seemed to understand my plight.

One suggested that it was OK for boys (but not for girls) to have sex by themselves, perhaps once a week—provided they didn't do it for pleasure. Well, that was no good. The only reason I did it was for the pleasant sensations, and particularly that fantastic 'orgasm' (climax) at the end. If I hadn't enjoyed it, I wouldn't have done it!

The other book told me that sex by myself was a poor substitute for the 'real thing', i.e. satisfying love-making in marriage. Well, thanks!! Adrian Mole in his *Secret Diary* can work that much out!

> Once again I am spotty. I am also extremely sexually frustrated. I'm sure a session of passionate love-making would improve my skin.
> Pandora says she is not going to risk being a single parent just for the sake of a few spots. So I will have to fall back on self-indulgence.[33]

My problem was that sex by myself seemed to be

114

my *only* alternative. As a Christian I was committed to no love-making outside marriage, and there was no likelihood of a marriage partner for several years. Far from being a 'second best', sex by myself appeared the one and only first best. So what was I supposed to do about it?

Most of the other books took what I call the 'traditional line'. They didn't go quite as far as Lord Baden-Powell, the founder of the Boy Scouts, but their vibes felt much the same as his!

> Some boys, like those who start smoking, think it is a very fine and manly thing to tell or listen to dirty stories, but it only shows them to be little fools. Yet such talk or the reading of trashy books or looking at lewd pictures are very apt to lead a thoughtless boy into the temptation of masturbation. This tends to lower both health and spirits. But if you have any manliness in you, you will throw off such temptation at once.[34]

Would that it were so easy! Lest you think that nobody these days could take such a black-and-white view, I should report that at the end of 1983 the Vatican restated the Roman Catholic teaching that masturbation (along with homosexuality and sex outside marriage) is 'a grave moral disorder, for which there is no justification'.

Put more sympathetically and more reasonably, the traditional line says that sex by yourself is wrong in God's sight because:

1. it is a selfish pleasure

2. it misuses God's gift of sexual release, intended for marriage

3. it becomes an enslaving habit, preventing you from growing up into more mature relationships

4. it involves lustful thoughts

5. it brings shame and guilt.

Therefore, the traditional line continues, you should ask for God's forgiveness and for his power to set you free from it. Meanwhile, help yourself as well by:

1. not getting it out of proportion—there are many worse sins and you needn't hate yourself for it

2. keeping yourself away from tempting sights or sounds which build up the pressure

3. keeping yourself busy with pure, healthy pursuits.

This view *may* be right. It may *well* be right for some people. For ten years I held it myself, and it contains a lot of sense. If it rings bells for you, and sounds the right way forward, please act on it. And read one of the fuller presentations of it in the books listed under endnote 35 at the back of this book. They are much more helpful than the books around in my young days. Then you can skip the rest of this chapter.

However (if you want to read on), I have a problem with the traditional view. It's not just that it didn't work for me. For out of well over a hundred people I've talked to about sex by yourself,

I've only met three for whom it has worked in any sense at all. And on closer examination, they are not much help to most teenagers. One of them says he got free when he was eighteen; another was twenty-four and already married(!); the third —a very unusual person—never had sex by himself, and therefore in a sense had nothing to be delivered from. The first two, I suspect, are typical of most boys, who do not 'grow out' of sex on their own until they are fully 'grown up'.

On the other hand, I have met many more than three who have given up being Christians and/or are angry against God because they tried praying and they could not shake free of having sex by themselves. They had understood that he promised to deliver them, but he didn't. Conclusion: *either* prayer, Christianity and God don't work, *or* I'm a total wash-out as a person.

One of them told me, 'I spent my teenage years in depression because I was told this was a sin, and yet I could get no "victory" over it. I decided I was no good as a Christian. Only now do I think that perhaps God was answering my prayers after all. I got no "victory over sin", *because it wasn't a sin!'*

This is the conclusion that I too have reached for myself. When I found myself a full-time missionary and still regularly having sex by myself, it was obviously necessary to get myself sorted out! This is how my thinking went.

First, it gradually sank in as a huge relief that I was not the only one. Virtually every teenage boy has sex by himself regularly at some stage. The old saying is: 'Nine out of ten boys admit they masturbate, and the tenth is a liar!' A lot of girls do too. Not all, by any means, for the reason we've already mentioned, that their sexual instincts are less immediately physical. Nonetheless, many do have sex by themselves—about sixty per cent of all teenage girls, according to one survey.[36]

Secondly, it does you no medical harm whatever. It doesn't make you go blind or bald or bats; it doesn't give you twitches, or ruin your married life! These are old scare stories on a par with the rot one Victorian father told his son: 'Your brain is full of grey matter, a kind of jelly. Touch yourself in that evil way and this jelly will leak down your spine and go to waste.'[37]

Thirdly, and much the most important, God nowhere says in the Bible, 'You mustn't have sex by yourself.' This is a subject on which he does not lay down the law.

There are many such subjects in Christian living. And they are not just 'modern' subjects which have only cropped up since the Bible was written, like abortion, euthanasia or nuclear weapons. God is 'silent', or at least not crystal clear, in the Bible about subjects that must have been important then, as they are now. Questions such as, 'Is it all right to drink alcohol in moderation?', 'Should you baptize the babies of Christian parents?', 'What is the best way to spend Sundays?' And another is, 'Is it OK to have sex by yourself?'

In Romans 14, Paul deals with two such questions that were troubling the early church: (1) whether to eat meat that had been offered in idol worship, and (2) whether to celebrate special festival days. He draws out several important principles that apply to all these questions of conscience, where God does not give specific instructions.

1. There are areas of life in which it is right to form personal opinions. Different Christians will reach different points of view. God's will for one person is not necessarily the same as his solution and provision for another. What is right for Christian A may be wrong for Christian B (verses 1–2).

2. We should respect, not condemn, those who take a different line from ours (verses 3–4).

3. We should not keep swerving in uncertainty from one interpretation to another, but firmly make up our own minds (verse 5).

4. Whatever decision we reach, and whatever action we take, should seek to honour Jesus as our King, and express our thanks to God (verses 6–9).

5. We must be ready to explain our choice to God, when he judges us at the end of the world (verses 10–12).

6. Don't do anything that will harm a fellow Christian (verses 13–21).

7. In the last resort, it is a matter between you and God; keep your conscience clear before him (verse 22).

8. If in doubt about anything, don't do it (verse 23)!

The impact of this and similar chapters on me was immense. The foundation truth I anchored on was that I must not say to myself or to anyone else that the act of sex on your own is a sin *in itself*.

God does not condemn it in his book. Occasionally people dispute this, and mutter something about Onan, but they are quite mistaken. The sad story of Onan occurs in Genesis 38:1–10. He came to a sticky end because he fell foul of the so-called 'levirate law'. This was a custom practised by Israel's neighbours, and approved by God at least for a stage of his people's development. The idea was that if a man died childless, it was his brother's duty to keep the family name going by marrying the widow and giving her children. (*Levir* is the Latin word for 'husband's brother', hence the name 'levirate'.)

This is what happened to Onan. But the snag in the system for him was that any children of this new relationship would count as Er's, not his; and as Er had been his elder brother, they would oust his own children from receiving the family inheritance. So he decided to prevent Tamar from becoming pregnant. He did this by repeated use of what is known as the 'withdrawal method' of contraception; that is, he withdrew his penis from her vagina before he reached his orgasm. (The Bible is not squeamish about these details!)

God punished him for this in the sharp way that he used when his people were still so few that their very survival was under threat. But what exactly did Onan do to displease him? The answer is that he disobeyed the levirate law, and in so doing cheated his family, his sister-in-law and the memory of his brother. It would be quite wrong to deduce from this story that contraception as such displeases God. Now that God has enabled us through hygiene and medicine to practise such effective 'death control', it is simply responsible to use some form of *birth* control in this crowded world.

It is even more wrong—and here we return to the subject of this chapter—to say that Onan was punished for having sex on his own. (But this misunderstanding is so persistent that 'onanism' is another name for masturbation.) Although he had his ejaculation by himself, and let his semen, or seed, fall on the floor of his tent, he quite clearly shared the rest of the sex act with Tamar. Nowhere else in the Bible comes as close as this to mentioning sex with yourself.

Because God does not condemn masturbation in his book, it would be out of step with God for me to condemn it. Jesus criticized the Pharisees and law-teachers of his day for inventing extra commands and taboos beyond what God requires (Matthew 23:4; Luke 11:46).

So why had I felt such guilt about it? My feelings of shame were, on reflection, partly man-made. There was undoubtedly a playback of being told off as a child for fiddling with my private parts—'It's just not nice!' And it took me a while to grow comfortable with the fact that the primary sexual sensations centre around what is also the urine exit! I now think this is a case both of God's brilliant economy of design, and of his sense of humour in keeping us from taking ourselves too seriously.

Then, to some extent, my 'guilt' was self-inflicted, and simply a symptom of wounded pride. I liked to think of myself as a strong character, able to resist the addictions that showed other people up as weaklings. I never smoked, and laughed at people who did. I didn't like alcohol, and scorned my friends who didn't seem to be able to enjoy life without their daily pint or three. To admit that *I*, puritanical, self-righteous me, was secretly hooked on a *sexual* habit was more than I could bear.

This was where my sense of shame mingled with fear of what others would think. My mother once caught me 'at it' (red-handed!); the anguish of that moment, and what it did to lower me in her opinion or would do to anyone else who knew about it, took years to work through.

My expectation of how other people regarded the practice was heavily influenced by my researches in the dictionary. One defined masturbation as 'self-abuse', another as 'self-pollution'! Both are highly loaded and unfair explanations. The word's origin is simply descriptive; it means 'disturbing your virile limb'!

But I can't pretend that all my feelings of guilt were only manward shame, and therefore not guilt at all. I'm sure there was an element of God-given guilty conscience mixed in there as well.

What I now came to see more clearly was that this was not on account of the physical actions themselves, but because of the thoughts that went with them.

Like most people, I used to fantasize while I had sex by myself. This is another ugly word, but it basically means the same as Jesus' words 'looking at a woman lustfully', which we thought about in the previous chapter. I *imagined* that I was not having sex on my own, but making love to someone I knew and desired; or I relived a bed-scene from a film, with me in the role of conquering hero!

Now *that* clearly was sin, as Jesus had taught. I needed to confess it, to receive forgiveness and to turn my back on it. But did it make all sex by myself sinful? Some words of Leslie Weatherhead struck me as relevant. Someone asked him, 'Is masturbation a sin?' and he answered, 'It depends whether the picture on the screen of the mind at the time could be shown to our Lord without shame.' That seems exactly right, in placing the responsibility for decision at the heart of the individual's relationship with Jesus.

And so, as I tried to reach an honest working arrangement with the Lord, the conversation seemed to me to go something like this.

> ME: Lord, if you can keep the TV screen of my mind clear of other people and wrong thoughts, I'd like to go ahead, free of guilt and shame.
> JESUS: But can you face the fact that I am there with you, watching?
> ME: Yes, Lord, *I* know *you* know what I'm doing. Forgive me for so often in the past pretending or

wishing you were out of the room.

JESUS: Are you ready to give account of the way you have used your body on the Day of Judgement?

ME: Yes, Lord. I believe this conversation is helping me to talk honestly and sensibly to you about what is important to me (and therefore important to you, because you love me and care for me).

JESUS: Can you honestly look me in the face and say thank you for what you're doing?

I thought long and hard about this one. And as I thought, the words of 1 Corinthians 10:31 (from another discussion of questions of conscience) kept ringing in my mind: 'Well, whatever you do, whether you eat or drink, do it all for God's glory.' God's glory? *Whatever* I do? Even *this*?! Could I possibly manhandle myself to God's glory?

At first the thought struck me as verging on blasphemy. But then I noticed the previous verse. As I read it, I substituted, as I had all along, 'sex' for 'food': 'If I thank God for my food [sex], why should anyone criticize me about food [sex] for which I give thanks?' Is thanking God for something the same as doing it to his glory? Well, it is certainly part of it—'Giving thanks is the sacrifice that honours me' (Psalm 50:23). So could I *honestly* thank Jesus to his face for sex by myself? My answer was ready.

ME: Yes, Lord. I thank you from the bottom of my heart that you have made me a bloke with these strong sexual feelings which I want to open up to you. And I thank you more than I can put into words for allowing me, as I see it, to cope in this way with the pressures on me—unless or until I get married.

And I *believe* from what I know of him (though of course I can't be sure), that as I looked him in the face, Jesus looked into mine with a smile of understanding and not a glare of disapproval.

So there. I had 'firmly made up [my] own mind', as instructed in Romans 14:5. I asked God to confirm it with the blessing of verse 22, if I had decided the right way: 'Happy is the person who does not feel guilty when he does something he judges is right!'

I can only state what I have found to be true: that I could then, and still can when separated from my wife, relieve sexual tension without lust. There is nobody else there in my thoughts. It is between me and God. I am intensely aware of his presence, and ceaselessly thank him for what I now see as this pure, healthy way of living with myself and staying faithful to him.

This has proved the biggest 'step up' in my growth as a Christian. My love for Jesus became much more close and personal for having got through the earlier blockage. And I became a much happier, more relaxed person as a result. And by one of those twists of human nature, once I saw sex by myself as something God trusted me to use responsibly in his presence, and no longer as the unmentionable vice, it stopped being a haunting compulsion. I actually had sex with myself less than before!

Now, all of that is just one person's experience.

I'm sorry to have laboured it at such length. But several people have said it has helped them work out their own way forward to hear someone cheeky enough to spell out his own thoughts and struggles.

You may be totally different. You may have found some of what I've said quite shocking, and decided (as if you hadn't already) that I'm a dangerous sex-maniac!

Well OK, I expect that reaction and I accept it. Remember, this is a subject on which people are rightly going to reach different opinions. I don't in the least want to force mine on you.

The question is, what is *your* attitude to sex by yourself? Have you tried to ignore it, and 'hope it will go away', or have you found God's plan *for you*? And are you peacefully, thankfully drawing on his love and strength to put it into practice?

7
Homosexuality

Shock Me, Doctor

I am not a normal man.
Cure me, doctor, if you can.
Banish by electric wire
My unnatural desire.

Flash those pictures on a screen,
Therapeutic but obscene;
When it is a naked girl
Wave a flag and ring a bell.

But if it should be a boy
Punish my Platonic joy
Shock me, doctor, through and through
Till I feel the same as you.

Turn my liking to disgust,
Fill me up with proper lust;
Wash my brain until I fit,
Make me think a miss a hit.[38]

By now you will be thinking, 'Surely this guy

can't have any *more* skeletons in his cupboard. He's confessed to just about everything already!' Well, there is just one more thing.

When I was seventeen (and still good-looking!), I could have used a book like this that tried to explain Christian ideas about sex. The only trouble with this particular book would have been that every chapter up to now would at some point have rubbed salt into the wound that made me feel different.

I spent a lot of time in my later teens feeling hopeless and depressed because my sexual feelings or instincts were what we call 'homosexual', not 'heterosexual'. Those are two long, ugly words, but in simple language they mean that I was attracted to other boys (homosexual) and not to girls (heterosexual).

Now I am a classic case of someone this was almost bound to happen to. I am the only child of divorced parents, and I was brought up by my mum in a one-parent family. To have, as I had, a thoroughly dominant mum (who had to do all the parenting), and a totally absent dad (or a dad who is ineffective in other ways), is a recipe for what's called 'sexual inversion'. That means 'turning in' —a bloke turns towards his own sex for friendship and sexual attraction, rather than out towards the opposite sex. And the same equation works in reverse for girls: an overassertive dad and a non-existent or downtrodden mum can push towards romantic feelings for other girls instead of boys.

It's perhaps easier to understand the effect of

the overbearing *opposite*-sex parent, than of the incomplete *same*-sex one. If a boy has been 's-mothered' all his life, you can understand him fearing that *all* women want to boss him around or gobble him up—not good for the male self-image! And if a girl has a cruel ogre of a Dad, she's going to need a lot of persuading that men are not always like that.

But recent evidence suggests that it is a failure in the relationship with your same-sex parent that is most likely to lead to homosexual feelings.[39] A child needs, as part of growing up, to feel attached to the parent most like him, and to copy him. A boy models himself on his daddy, and a girl imagines herself as her mummy.

Now, if that parent is unsatisfactory or removed, a vital part of growing up is blocked. And teenage love for a fellow boy or girl can often be a late discovery of a replacement parent-figure or childhood same-sex friend. The emotional need it meets is not at root physical. But it takes on sexual attraction as well, because it comes at the moment when sexual feelings are at their noisiest! If this evidence is right, male homosexuality is likely to increase with the growing number of single-parent families and children not knowing who their dad really is.

My case was more complicated still. I went to a boys' boarding school, then an all-male college. And the first two jobs I had were also in single-sex institutions.

It stands to reason that if you deprive men of any female company, their eyes will rove *either* to page three of *The Sun* (at least!) *or* to the most girlish looking of their companions. The armed forces and prisons understandably report a higher than average frequency of homosexuality for this reason.

But quite apart from sob stories like mine, the nearest we can get to statistics in this extremely personal area suggests that same-sex attraction is common, even when there are no obvious family or environmental causes. Probably one out of every three boys passes through, during his teens, however briefly, a phase when he finds other boys more attractive than girls. No one seems to have worked out how many girls this happens to, but there are certainly some.

Among adults, it seems that one in perhaps twenty or twenty-five still feel their sexual leanings in the direction of their own sex. This would total about 2½ million people in Britain, roughly equivalent to the population of Wales. So it's likely that between a quarter and a third of you who read this book will know what I'm talking about, even if only from memory. But even if you've never felt the slightest homosexual tremor, stick around till the end of the chapter, because I'm as much concerned with how other people react to homosexuals, as I am with how homosexuals understand themselves.

The problem comes in knowing how to obey God's teaching in the Bible and live it out. There are not many references to homosexuality—seven definite ones, all told. One thing is clear, though —they all speak of homosexual intercourse or lust with disapproval.

Genesis 19 is the origin of the words 'sodomite' and 'sodomy'. The entire male population of Sodom tried to have sex with two male guests, who happened to be angels. As a judgement, the men were struck blind, and then God destroyed the city.

It is quite unfair to call *all* homosexual activity 'sodomy', because clearly what was in mind here was gang homosexual rape. (Who said the Bible was irrelevant in the age of video-nasties?!) A curiously similar incident occurred hundreds of years later in Gibeah, recorded in Judges 19. The outcome was even more horrific, because this time God did not step in. The man who was the target of the townsfolk's lust sent his mistress out to them instead. Evidently, they had no strong preference over male or female, for 'they raped her and abused her all night long and didn't stop until morning' (Judges 19:25), when she collapsed and died.

The law-code in Leviticus twice forbids male homosexual intercourse in the strongest terms: 'No man is to have sexual relations with another man; God hates that' (Leviticus 18:22); 'If a man has sexual relations with another man, they have done a disgusting thing, and both shall be put to death' (Leviticus 20:13). Quoted on their own, these prohibitions outlaw homosexual relations pretty comprehensively. But the setting is largely concerned with congregational worship, and the ban *may* be focused on male temple-prostitutes, common in the Canaanite shrines that Moses was now preparing to 'clean up'. It is impossible to be absolutely certain whether these laws are condemning *any* male homosexual intercourse, or the practice of performing it in public in services of worship.

When we come to the New Testament, there is only one *discussion* on the subject, and two further *mentions*. All come from the apostle Paul.

The discussion is in Romans 1. In the second half of that chapter, he explains how God shows his anger at human sin. Because people refuse to worship him as Creator, and insist on idolizing parts of his creation, he 'gives them over' to the consequences of their rebellious choice.

The first example he gives, and the only one he examines in detail, is homosexual activity:

> Because they do this, God has given them over to shameful passions. Even the women pervert the natural use of their sex by unnatural acts. In the same way the men give up natural sexual relations with women and burn with passion for each other. Men do shameful things with each other, and as a result they bring upon themselves the punishment they deserve for their wrongdoing (Romans 1:26–27).

There are various things to say about this. Paul may place homosexual acts at the top of his list of sins (the rest are in verses 29–31) partly because, as we have seen, sexuality is so basic to our human nature. Partly, too, it may be because it was such a common vice in the ancient world. Fourteen of the first fifteen Roman emperors were practising homosexuals. Nero, who was almost certainly Emperor when Paul wrote this letter, publicly married *both* a boy-wife (Sporus) *and* (this time casting himself in the female role) a husband (Pythagoras—same name as the famous mathematician, but not the same person).

Romans 1 is the only specific reference in the Bible to female homosexuality, or 'lesbianism' as it is often called (after the Greek island of Lesbos, where the seventh century BC poetess, Sappho, is said to have encouraged the practice). This does not mean that girls' homosexuality is less important to God than boys'. Paul's wording seems to suggest that God regards both sexes alike ('In the same way. . .'), and perhaps that lesbianism is even more grievous to him ('Even the women. . .').

At first sight, Paul seems to be following the Old Testament references in talking about what is technically known as homosexual *perversion*. This means people who are by nature heterosexual (attracted to the opposite sex), experimenting with unnatural homosexual acts for kicks. This sounds like the obvious sense of 'the women pervert the natural use of their sex by unnatural acts' and 'men give up natural sexual relations with women and . . . do shameful things with each other.' On balance, I *think* it is what Paul had in mind.

But it is possible that Paul is not so much thinking of *particular* people spicing up their sex life with homosexual variations, as commenting on a *general* trend in human behaviour. In this case, he will mean that the very existence of homosexual activity in the world perverts or twists the natural man-woman sexuality that God designed.

Some people use the first, more particular interpretation of Romans 1:26–27, alongside the Old Testament passages, to argue that the Bible nowhere forbids love-making between *inverts,* i.e. people who are homosexual by nature and who would find heterosexual intercourse 'unnatural'. But Paul's other two mentions of homosexual acts contradict this argument, even if the Good News Bible translation makes them sound as if they don't!

The first is 1 Corinthians 6:9–10, where the Good News Bible totally fails to do justice to what Paul wrote. It reads: 'Surely you know that the wicked will not possess God's kingdom. Do not fool yourselves; people who are immoral or who worship idols or are adulterers or *homosexual perverts* . . . none of these will possess God's king-dom' (my italics).

But here are some more Greek words for you to 'enjoy'! Paul actually lists, after 'adulterers', two groups of people: *malakoi* and *arsenokoitai*(!) *Malakoi* means soft or effeminate, and was the Greek equivalent of our slang 'fairy' or 'queen'; it means the male 'woman', the man on the receiving end of homosexual intercourse. And *arseno-koitai* means, as you may have guessed, people having *coitus* or intercourse with men, i.e., the 'male' or 'wooing' partner when two men sleep together.

In other words, Paul describes an act of homo-sexual intercourse, and says, 'That does not happen in God's kingdom. You cannot go to bed with a same-sex partner, *whether or not you love them,* and claim to be acting under Jesus' lordship.'

He says much the same thing in 1 Timothy 1: 9–10, where again the Good News Bible is misleading.

> It must be remembered, of course, that laws are made, not for good people, but for lawbreakers and criminals, for the godless and sinful, for those who are not religious or spiritual, for those who kill their fathers or mothers, for murderers, for the immoral, for *sexual perverts*. . . (my italics).

But Paul's word is once again *arsenokoitai*, which simply means men having homosexual intercourse, and makes no pronouncement on whether their motive is *per*verted or *in*verted.

In both 1 Corinthians and 1 Timothy, Paul links homosexual activity with some pretty gruesome bedfellows (if you'll pardon the expression) —stealing, drunkenness, murder, kidnap, lying. The point he is making to Timothy is that God's law forbids and condemns these things.

And even if the law, in the sense of Old Testament commandments, does not, as we have seen, legislate against *all* homosexual practice very clearly or very often, it is a fair deduction from the all-important 'Maker's Handbook' in Genesis 1 and 2. You will remember that God says there that he designed man for woman, and elementary anatomy shows what he meant, in comparing the male and female physical shapes! It is perfectly reasonable to add that he did *not* design man to belong to man, or woman to woman—their bodies just don't fit!

So, to sum up, God definitely rules out homosexual lust, rape, prostitution and perverted experiments. They are as wrong as heterosexual lust, rape and prostitution, or any other form of 'kinky', twisted sex. But he also by implication seems to rule out any homosexual intercourse or stroking of the genital organs to climax. And he does this in order to keep safe for us his garden of delights—man-woman marriage.

Homosexual sin is as wrong as any other sexual sin, or, more bluntly, as *any* other sin. But it is no worse. Yet there is a lingering suspicion that homosexuality is somehow the unforgivable sin. The Emperor Justinian (one Roman emperor who *did* have worries on the subject!) thought homosexuality was the cause of earthquakes! And people throughout history have taught that homosexuality leads to the breakdown of civilization. There may be sociological reasons for believing this, but there are none that I can see in the Bible.

Shortly after I became a Christian, a Church of England bishop publicly suggested that perhaps Jesus was a homosexual because he never married. There is not a shred of evidence for this idea, which should be most politely dismissed as sheer imagination. But equally there is no excuse for some of the reactions it provoked. I vividly remember a visiting preacher naming out loud the offending bishop for 'accusing my Saviour of the vilest sin there is'. We shall think later a little more about why he found it so revolting. But enough to say for now that homosexual activity is *not* the vilest sin there is. Jesus specifically taught that the sins of Chorazin, Bethsaida and Capernaum (rejecting him) are *worse* than the sin of Sodom (Matthew 11:20–24). Where the Bible calls homosexual behaviour sin, it ranks alongside random lists of other sins.

So if this is where you are tempted and sore, you can come out from under that cloud of worry and fear. Your temptation and sin (if there has been sin) are no worse, nor any better, than my pride, jealousy and untruthfulness.

Your help, as with any other sin, lies in Jesus. As we have just seen, he knows what it is like to be *called* a homosexual. And as ever, he offers his forgiveness for wrongdoing and his strength for right living.

I urge you, as your friend and brother, to take very great care indeed not to get involved in a homosexual affair. Not only does God say 'don't', but the law of the land also makes it illegal for anyone under the age of twenty-one. This is one area where the official age of adulthood has not been lowered, and I think that was a wise decision.

Events of the last few years have proved it wiser than the legislators realized at the time. For since 1982 there has emerged the scare about AIDS. The letters stand for Acquired Immune Deficiency Syndrome, which in simple English means a disease that leaves you unable to recover from other diseases. At the moment anyone who catches it dies within months; but medical research will almost certainly discover how to cure and prevent it in due course.

Knowledge is still sketchy about how the disease is caught. But at least one way is through the blood, so rigorous tests are in force to prevent blood donors passing it on. Two known ways in which the bloodstream can be infected are: (1) injecting drugs with dirty syringes, and (2) male homosexual intercourse with someone already infected.

The number of people carrying the disease in Britain is small, but multiplying fast. If you have had sex with a boy or man you know or think is a practising homosexual, you would be wise to check with your doctor. Or if that would be too embarrassing, you can make an appointment at a hospital clinic—look up 'venereal diseases' in your local telephone directory to find the nearest one. When I talk of 'having sex with a boy', I mean full sexual intercourse with a sexually developed and experienced teenager. There is no danger of AIDS from playing around as a child, or from the first experiments of someone who has had sex with no one else.

But quite apart from the physical danger of AIDS, a homosexual encounter can leave a permanent psychological mark on those involved. Some who have fluttered with homosexuality for a laugh have found themselves scarred for life. A casual action can very easily become a habit, and then in turn a natural way of thought.

This seems to be a further angle of Paul's teaching in Romans 1:26–27: 'God has given them over to shameful *passions* ... men give up natural sexual relations with women and *burn with passion for each other*' (my italics). What starts as an outward experiment can become an all-consuming inward appetite.

Virtually all the Bible's teaching on homosexuality concentrates on physical actions. Except here, it does not talk directly about inner feelings. Obviously, when it does not overstep into burning lust, people cannot help a basic homosexual 'condition' or 'attraction'. Some people simply do prefer the look and the appeal of their own gender, and God does not blame them for it. In itself, it is as 'neutral' as being left-handed or having red hair; though in terms of handicap, a more complete comparison is with being an orphan or having a leg amputated.

For in at least one respect, it is as crippling as these misfortunes. In Matthew 19:12 Jesus teaches that some 'men cannot marry: some, because they were born that way; others, because men made them that way. . . .' Almost certainly he has other reasons in mind as well; other pressures from 'the way they are' or from what life has done to them, that makes some people unsuited to marriage. Some of these pressures are physical, some mental, some emotional. But one of them seems likely to be a homosexual condition ('born that way'), or experience ('men made them that way').

For people who are genuinely and lastingly homosexual, marriage is not on unless they find, as some do, an understanding opposite-sex spouse. This is desperately hard to face up to, but not really any harder than for heterosexuals who find themselves unable to marry, for whatever reason. And Jesus sweetens the pill by saying *twice* (verses 11 and 12) that where God calls, he enables. 'This teaching does not apply to everyone, but only to those to whom God has *given* it' (my italics). Singleness, for whatever reason, is God's gift, designed to fit that person. When he asks you to do something unusual, he gives the strength to make it possible. That's the good news we need to help face the future.

And here's some more good news. If you've got homosexual feelings now, you're unlikely to have them all your life. Try to understand what is probably happening to you. When our sexual feelings first come alive, some of us can't 'make the jump' of latching them onto members of the opposite sex straightaway. So we start by focusing them on someone we feel closer to, and whom we understand better—a fellow boy or girl. Sometimes it is a distant hero-figure, whom we have a crush on from afar. Sometimes, as with me, it is someone younger, in whom we see echoes of ourselves and about whom we feel protective. Sometimes it is a close friend of the same age. Even when they return the feeling, this attraction need not turn into sexual activity; it often remains at the level of gentle, caring devotion.

Provided these feelings are kept in line with God's loving guidance, they can be an important, formative first stage in learning to be less shy, and in beginning to project that sexual longing out towards the other sex; and, God permitting and in his good time, to the one particular member of the other sex he has planned for us.

In fact virtually nobody is 100% homosexual or 100% heterosexual. We are all our own unique mixture of feelings. What happens to some people in their teens is that they move from being mostly homosexual to mostly heterosexual. Sometimes it takes only a few weeks, sometimes months, sometimes, as in my case, years. But I praise God that that is what happened to me, under his loving care.

Working on mixed teams at Christian holiday ventures, I came to know a number of Christian girls. And it gradually dawned on me that many of them were very caring and gentle. I lost my fear of being henpecked! And so I became more able to form good friendships with them, instead of being paralysed with shyness as I had been before.

It was around this time that a Christian magazine ran an anonymous survey on attitudes to women's ministry in the church. I decided I was all in favour. This was just as well, as my future wife was already training to be a full-time deaconess! As my final comment on the form I wrote, 'Girls are gorgeous, and God made them so!'

The magazine described it as 'a light-hearted remark from a bachelor in his thirties'! They did not realize the years of struggle and very gradual progress that lay behind it. In fact, their comment was spot on in one sense—my heart was indeed light and free. That one sentence had signalled my liberation into the sexual 'orientation' or direction, that God intended.

So if you are going through a 'mainly homosexual stage' in your thoughts and feelings, it is vital not to think of yourself as a 'homosexual'. Your sexual identity is still unfixed in your teens, and you'll almost certainly move forwards soon if you keep your eyes on the goal of Emmanuel-sex: marriage with a partner of the opposite sex, when God's time comes.

Of course, if you *do* find yourself stuck for a long time, or if you are into more complicated distortions, such as wanting to be or to dress like a member of the opposite sex, you need trained help and one form or another of God's healing power—and you can find it. Start by asking your minister or doctor or someone else you trust. If you don't know any one you could talk to face to face, write to the True Freedom Trust, P.O. Box 3, Upton, Wirral, L49 6NY. They will either help you by correspondence or put you in touch with a sympathetic friend near where you live.

But please, whoever you are, don't stick the label 'gay' on somebody else, unless they positively ask you to. It is a nicer word than 'queer', but in my experience homosexuals are very seldom gay in the 'straight' sense of the word. Some adults achieve a sense of pride in coming to terms with their own feelings. But for teenagers it is a bitterly frustrating state to be in, usually made much worse by the attitudes of the rest of us.

You can feel some of the pain of the condition

itself in the poem at the start of this chapter.
Despite the jokey tone, the male patient is talking
about unpleasant electric-shock treatment, intended to reprogram his sexual desires so that he
learns to be 'turned on' by pictures of girls rather
than boys. The success rate of this and other
psychiatric treatment is very uncertain. And
prayer for healing, we have to admit from experience, is similarly not guaranteed to produce an
instant change.

A basically homosexual orientation can feel
desperately stubborn. It calls for sympathetic
understanding, not for jokes and jeers. The
instinct of horror and disgust in heterosexuals at
the thought of homosexuality is partly irrational,
partly understandable. The inconsistent, purely
Anglo-Saxon part is the way in which two girls are
allowed to kiss in a public place as a matter of
form. But if two boys flung their arms round one
another . . . can't you hear the shocked comments
from some quarters? Yet Frenchmen and
Russians can apparently embrace each other without giving anyone a fit!

The more understandable revulsion at homosexuality is probably a deep human drive to resist
anything which threatens the continued existence
of the race. And often people have a subconscious
fear (which may be well grounded, as we have
seen) that they are not as securely 'normal' themselves as they would like to think.

But understandable as these instincts are,
Christians must not allow them to spill over into
their treatment of those who are homosexually

inclined. It is really heartbreaking when Christians—the people who are meant to be following Jesus—shut homosexuals out, or call them 'poofs' to their faces. I often think that the harsh, condemning attitude of some Christians must pain Jesus more than any homosexual sins they are judging.

Homosexuals have received the most blood-curdling persecution from the Christian church throughout history. Do you know why homosexuals are sometimes called 'fags'? Because in the Middle Ages they were publicly burnt as human 'fagots' or firewood. We owe them a massive debt of prayer, care and help.

One way we can help is to show that *we* are not prejudiced anti-homosexuals. 'Queer' is so much the thing *not* to be in most circles, that its victims have to add secrecy to all their other burdens. It can be a huge relief simply to discover from someone's attitudes and conversation that they don't regard homosexuals as if they had some infectious disease.

And another way we can help is by being friends. As we saw earlier, many people in a homosexual phase are looking for the close friend that their same-sex parent wasn't. They don't really want a sexual partner so much as a trusting, sharing companion or group of companions to see them through this bumpy part of growing up. We ought to make it public knowledge that the place to look for real, caring friendship is among the friends of Jesus. Often this warm, open love will help someone grow through the homosexual inclinations 'unconsciously', without anyone else realizing what is happening.

It would, though, be a good test of your church or youth fellowship to see whether a member knows that he or she could say to one or more of you (if he or she wants to), 'Look, I'd like you to pray for me, because I'm troubled by homosexual thoughts,' and still be as much loved, valued and trusted as before—if not more so. What a great chance to be part of the Lord's comforting, re-assuring, healing love for that boy or girl!

Our calling as Christians in our sexual attitudes, as in every other part of life, is to follow Jesus. And can you imagine Jesus responding to a cry of distress in any other way than, 'Son, Daughter, your faith is making you well. Come, join these others in following me'? I can't.

8

Rape or Rapture?

Portrait of a Young Girl Raped at a Suburban Party

And after this quick bash in the dark
You will rise and go
Thinking of how empty you have grown
And of whether all the evening's care in
    front of mirrors
And the younger boys disowned
Led simply to this.

Confined to what you are expected to be
By what you are
Out in this frozen garden
You shiver and vomit—
Frightened, drunk among trees,
You wonder at how those acts that called for
    tenderness
Were far from tender.

Now you have left your titterings about love
And your childishness behind you
Yet still far from being old
You spew up among flowers

And in the warm stale rooms
The party continues.

It seems you saw some use in moving away
From that group of drunken lives
Yet already ten minutes pregnant
In twenty thousand you might remember
This party
This dull Saturday evening
When planets rolled out of your eyes
And splashed down in suburban grasses.[40]

Last week, a twenty-year-old girl I know was viciously raped by three young men who broke into her home to burgle it. Yesterday the crime figures for 1985 were announced. Reported incidence of rape in the UK was up by 29% on the previous year.

Rape must surely be the most horrifying distortion of what God designed sex to be. A man (or men) force sexual entry into a woman against her will. Instead of expressing tenderness and love, sex is here a weapon of violence and hate. The experience can sometimes leave her a nervous wreck for life.

There may be many doors at which the blame could be laid for the rising tide of rape. But chief among them is surely Emmanuelle. She has encouraged men to measure their manliness by the score of their sexual conquests. She has driven them to lust for the sexual act as an achievement in its own right. She has placarded naked female bodies before their eyes as so many scalps to collect. She has told them that the girl's feelings hardly enter into the matter.

That's what she's up to, and I think it's high time that, in Emmanuel's name, we stopped her. Christians can press for rapists to receive just punishment for their savagery, and they should be in the forefront of caring for the victims of rape. But that is only half the battle. Let's get out there and recover every facet of sexual behaviour for Jesus.

We'll only succeed if we try a new approach. For centuries, the church has replied to Emmanuelle with an embarrassed, 'No sex, please, we're Christians.' This has simply played into her hands and proved her point. Now is the time to surprise both her and the world that believes her by shouting and living—a loud *yes!* 'Yes, sex pleases us Christians. Our Father invented it.'

Of course, we say no to the things that hurt and maim—selfishness, child abuse, pornography, unhelpful fantasies, sex without love, prostitution, adultery, divorce and rape. But only because they take us away from God's loving plan—the plan we say yes to.

Yes to the glory of being human—made like God, to be loved by God and love him in return.

Yes to being girl or boy, whichever he chose—thanks for the range and richness of my sexuality.

Yes to sex as the beautiful, funny, exciting way God devised to bring the two halves together and keep the race going.

Yes to God's law drawn up to protect me; the rules to help us win in the game of sex.

Yes to love—God's 'gut feeling' towards all other people, growing deeper in me towards those in need, especially any with sexual heartaches.

Yes to the warm sexual feelings in me—attraction and longing, hope and dream.

Yes to marriage as the perfect provision for people's social and sexual needs, the route God planned to sexual rapture.

Yes to God's will for my life now, bringing contentment and peace.

Yes to his promise to look after the future, saving me from worry and fret.

Yes to the tough, bracing challenge to learn self-control in a world largely out of control.

Yes to Jesus, King of love, who invites us, his church, to marry him. What rapture that will be!

> Let us rejoice and be glad; let us praise his greatness! For the time has come for the wedding of the Lamb, and his bride has prepared herself for it. The Spirit and the Bride say, 'Come!'
>
> He who gives his testimony to all this says, 'Yes indeed! I am coming soon!'
>
> So be it. Come, Lord Jesus! (Revelation 19:7; 22: 17, 20).

Notes

1. Steve Turner, *Up to Date* (London, Hodder and Stoughton, 1983), p.20.
2. I owe the inspiration for the Emmanuel–Emmanuelle concept (and for much else besides) to Prebendary Michael Saward, Vicar of Ealing. Those who have heard him or read his books will trace his influence throughout this book in its attempt to say thank you to God for sex. All the book's failings, on the other hand, are my fault, not his.
3. Quoted in Paul Dickson, *The Official Explanations* (London, Arrow Books, 1981), p.44.
4. John Pearson, *The Life of Ian Fleming* (London, Jonathan Cape), p.86.
5. Walter Trobisch, *Love Yourself* (Kehl-Rhein, West Germany, Editions Trobisch, 1976), p.5.
6. Michael Schofield, *The Sexual Behaviour of Young People* (Harlow, Longmans, 1965).
7. Alan Watts, *Beyond Theology; the Art of Godmanship* (New York, Random House, 1973).
8. Nanette Newman, *The Facts of Love* (London,

Collins, 1980).

9. N. F. Simpson, *One Way Pendulum* (London, Faber and Faber, 1960) pp.44–45.

10. Sue Townsend, *The Secret Diary of Adrian Mole, Aged 13¾* (London, Methuen, 1982), p.109.

11. Nanette Newman, *Lots of Love* (London, Collins, 1974).

12. Nanette Newman, *The Facts of Love* (London, Collins, 1980).

13. W. S. Gilbert, *Princess Ida* (Macmillan, London, 1957), p.226.

14. Eric Marshall and Stuart Hample, *Children's Letters to God* (London, Fount, 1977).

15. Albert Chevalier and Charles Ingle, *My Old Dutch* (EMI Publishing, 1911).

16. Arthur Miller, *The Crucible* (London, Heineman Educational Books, 1956), p.50.

17. George Bernard Shaw, *Man and Superman* (London, Penguin, 1908), p.274.

Martin Luther, quoted in Gyles Brandreth, *The Complete Husband* (London, Sidgwick and Jackson, 1978), p.268.

G. K. Chesterton, quoted in Derek Williams, *About People* (Leicester, Inter-Varsity Press, 1977), p.56.

George Eliot, *Adam Bede* (London, J. M. Dent, 1906), p.510.

Gloria Okes Perkins, quoted in Ed and Gaye Wheat, *Intended for Pleasure* (London, Scripture Union, 1979), p.206.

18. Based on research by Dr Nancy Clatworthy for *Seventeen* magazine, quoted in John Stott, *Issues Facing Christians Today* (Basingstoke, Marshall Morgan & Scott, 1984), pp.55–56.

19. Richard and Helen Exley, *What Is A Husband?* (Watford, Exley Publications, 1977), pp.4, 6, 14, 16, 22, 29.

20. R. A. Knox, *Bridegroom and Bride* (London, Sheed and Ward, 1957), p.26.

21. C. S. Lewis, *Mere Christianity* (London, Collins, 1952), p.99.

22. Michael Green, *Choose Freedom* (Leicester, Inter-Varsity Press, 1965), p.69.

23. Nanette Newman, *The Facts of Love* (London, Collins, 1980).

24. Halcyon Backhouse, 'Boyfriends', poem in *Teaching 10–13s* magazine (Scripture Union).

25. Sue Townsend, *The Secret Diary of Adrian Mole, Aged 13¾* (London, Methuen, 1982), p.187.

26. Stephen Pile, *The Book of Heroic Failures* (London, Routledge and Kegan Paul, 1979), p.128.

27. Nanette Newman, *Lots of Love* (London, Collins, 1974).

28. Walter Trobisch, *Love Is A Feeling To Be Learned* (Kehl-Rhein, West Germany, Editions Trobisch 1971), p.5.

29. Lyman Coleman and Denny Rydberg, *Front Line* (London, Scripture Union, 1984), p.14.

30. Nanette Newman, *Lots of Love* (London, Collins, 1974).

31. Norman C. Habel, *Interrobang* (Guildford, Lutterworth, 1970), pp.44–45.

32. Michael Schofield, *The Sexual Behaviour of Young People* (London, Longmans, 1965).

33. Sue Townsend, *The Secret Diary of Adrian Mole, Aged 13¾* (London, Methuen, 1982), p.176.

34.   Robert Baden-Powell, *Scouting for Boys* (C. Arthur Pearson, 1932).

35.   Joyce Huggett, *Just Good Friends?* chapter 10 (Leicester, Inter-Varsity Press, 1985); Walter and Ingrid Trobisch, *My Beautiful Feeling* (Kehl-Rhein, West Germany, Editions Trobisch, 1975); John White, *Eros Defiled*, chapter 4 (Leicester, Inter-Varsity Press, 1977).

36.   Walter R. Johnson, *Siecus Study Guide Number 3: Masturbation* (Sex Information and Education Council of the United States, 1968), p.7.

37.   Thomas Blackburn, *'A Clip of Steel'*, reviewed by Arthur Marshall, *Girls will be Girls* (London, Hamish Hamilton, 1974), p.146.

38.   Sydney Carter, *The Two-way Clock* (London, Stainer and Bell, 1974), p.121.

39.   Elizabeth R. Moberly, *Homosexuality: A New Christian Ethic* (Cambridge, James Clarke, 1983), p.146.

40.   Brian Patten, *Notes to the Hurrying Man* (London, Allen and Unwin).

Suggested Reading

Joyce Huggett, *Growing into Love* (Leicester, Inter-Varsity Press, 1982). A practical guide for engaged couples and those thinking of getting engaged.

Joyce Huggett, *Just Good Friends?* (Leicester, InterVarsity Press, 1985). A very thorough discussion of growing in relationships for the student generation.

Michael Lawson and Dr David Skipp, *Sex and That* (Tring, Lion, 1985). Basic facts and answers for young teenagers from a doctor and a counsellor. Very reassuring.

Herbert J. Miles, *Sexual Understanding before Marriage* (Grand Rapids, MI., Zondervan, 1971). An older American book for students, with emphasis on the biological aspects.

Michael Saward, *And So To Bed?* (Good Reading, 1975). The first English Christian book that tried to sound happy about sex. It makes you excited to be human and sexual!

Ulrich Schaffer, *Love Reaches Out* (Tring, Lion,

1976). Meditations for people in love.

Charles W. Shedd, *The Stork is Dead* (Waco, Texas, Word Books, 1968). Out of print now, but well worth looking for on your youth leader's or minister's bookshelves. Wise answers to letters received while the author wrote a weekly column for America's *TEEN Magazine*.

Walter Trobisch, *Love Yourself* (Kehl-Rhein, West Germany, Editions Trobisch, 1976). A short aid to self-acceptance and overcoming depression as a step to building relationships with others.